'This beautifully wrought, multi-layered, multiv imprint of the "war experience" in Ukraine: on the ᴜᴏᴅʏ ᴀᴜᴅ ᴛᴜᴇ soul, on sense and memory (collective and singular), on knowing and unknowing, on loss, care, ruin, and survival. It challenges the very notion of trauma's "inability to be represented" by taking the time to dwell in the lived realities and dreamscapes of civilians for whom war is an enduring experience. Drawing upon visual, personal, philosophical, and historiographic approaches, the contributors paint for us a complex yet intimate portrait of people facing precarity and violence who, nonetheless and despite, remain in place.'

Jeanne Morefield, *Associate Professor at the Department of Politics and International Relations, University of Oxford, UK*

'*Psychosocial and Cultural Perspectives on the War in Ukraine: Imprints and Dreamscapes* brings together diaries, testimonies, visual material documenting the war and its effects on an individual life. This raw material of war is set in the elaborated analytical framework that draws on psychoanalysis, philosophy, sociology, and cultural studies and helps the readers to understand the workings of war through the human existence. A powerful book which will leave a haunting and unforgettable imprint in anyone who reads it.'

Yuliya Yurchuk, *Assistant Professor at Södertörn University, Sweden*

'This is a deeply moving and highly relevant collection. It is good to see nuanced thought in these troubling times.'

Astrid Erll, *Professor at Goethe University Frankfurt and The Frankfurt Memory Studies Platform, Germany*

PSYCHOSOCIAL AND CULTURAL PERSPECTIVES ON THE WAR IN UKRAINE

This innovative and important book explores how war imprints on culture and the psychosocial effects of war on individuals and societies, based on the first few months after the outbreak of war in Ukraine in 2022.

The book approaches the conflict in Ukraine through the prism of creative and artistic material alongside scholarly analysis to highlight the multiplicity of subjective experiences. Essays are complemented by material from the 'war diaries', which comprise day diaries, dream diaries, artistic and poetic material composed by students and academics in February and March 2022. With chapters focusing on fear, ruptures and resistance, the book examines different aspects of subjective, cultural and embodied experiences of war. It examines elements that dominant perspectives of war often overlook; the quotidian, personal and emotive ways that war is registered individually and collectively in societies and cultures.

Highlighting different narratives that illuminate the complex effects of war, this book is highly relevant for postgraduate students, researchers and advanced undergraduate students in the fields of cultural psychology, psychosocial studies, peace and conflict studies and cultural history.

Bohdan Shumylovych is an Associate Professor of Cultural Studies at the Ukrainian Catholic University. He also works at the Center for Urban History in Lviv, Ukraine.

Magdalena Zolkos is an Associate Professor in the Department of Social Sciences and Philosophy at the University of Jyväskylä, Finland.

PSYCHOSOCIAL AND CULTURAL PERSPECTIVES ON THE WAR IN UKRAINE

Imprints and Dreamscapes

Edited by Bohdan Shumylovych and Magdalena Zolkos

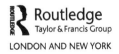

LONDON AND NEW YORK

Designed cover image: Anastasiia B. (2022). Untitled image.

First published 2024
by Routledge
4 Park Square, Milton Park, Abingdon, Oxon OX14 4RN

and by Routledge
605 Third Avenue, New York, NY 10158

Routledge is an imprint of the Taylor & Francis Group, an informa business

Funded by University of Jyväskylä, Magdalena Zolkos' Starting Grant

Trademark notice: Product or corporate names may be trademarks or registered
trademarks, and are used only for identification and explanation without intent
to infringe.

British Library Cataloguing-in-Publication Data
A catalogue record for this book is available from the British Library

ISBN: 978-1-032-58224-5 (hbk)
ISBN: 978-1-032-58219-1 (pbk)
ISBN: 978-1-003-44909-6 (ebk)

DOI: 10.4324/9781003449096

Typeset in Sabon
by MPS Limited, Dehradun

CONTENTS

Acknowledgements   *x*
Notes on Academic Contributors   *xii*
List of Contributions to Diaries of War and Life   *xvi*
List of Images (1): Drawings   *xviii*
List of Images (2): Photographs   *xix*

Introduction   1
Bohdan Shumylovych and Magdalena Zolkos

PART I
Recording Lived Experiences of War through Diaries,
Images and Dreams   **9**

1 Collective Practice of Meditation and Phenomenology
   of Consciousness in War   11
   Ihor Kolesnyk

2 'The Production of Fireflies': Searching for Truth and
   Truthfulness in the Diaries and Images of War,
   Conversation with Bohdan Shumylovych   22
   Bohdan Shumylovych and Magdalena Zolkos

3 The Emotional and Psychological Registers of
War: Conversation with Natalka Ilchyshyn   36
*Bohdan Shumylovych, Magdalena Zolkos,
and Natalka Ilchyshyn*

Excerpts from *Diaries of War and Life* (1)   43

PART II
The Ruptures and Ruins of War   **99**

4 Dreaming of War   101
Stephen Frosh

5 *'The Word Remains'*: War Diaries in
Ruptured Time and Space   117
Magda Schmukalla

6 The Image in Ruins   131
Martta Heikkilä

7 Quiet Trauma and the War in Ukraine   162
Chari Larsson

Excerpts from *Diaries of War and Life* (2)   196

PART III
Resistance, Endurance, Testimony   **249**

8 Unexpected Shapes of Courage:
Emotions of Resistance in Ukraine   251
Marguerite La Caze

9 The Determination to Resist: *Dumky* by
Young Ukrainians   261
Luisa Passerini

10 Testimony, Endurance, *Tryvoga*: A History
    Open to Shivering Bodies   274
    Magdalena Zolkos

Index   *287*

ACKNOWLEDGEMENTS

This project began as a collaboration between Bohdan Shumylovych, Ihor Kolesnyk and Natalka Ilyshyn in the early days following the full-scale invasion of Ukraine in February 2022. Bohdan, Ihor and Natalka brought together and inspired a group of Ukrainian students to create unique narrative and visual records of their lived experiences of war. The greatest thanks go to the participants in the project: Anastasiia B., Yelyzaveta B., Iryna B., Olena C., Oksana D., Sofia D., Mariana H., Oksana H., Anastasiia I., Anastasiia K., Anna K., Dana K., Ihor K., Mariia K., Miia K., Oksana K., Olha K., Stefaniia K., Kateryna L., Anastasiia M., Khrystia M., Yevheniia M., Daryna P., Oleksandra P., Kateryna R., Ruta R., Anna-Mariia S., Bohdan S., Polina S., Sofia S., Annamaria T., Zhenia T., Oksana V. and Viktoria Y., and those who contributed visual material: Eva Alvor, Anastasiia B., Lena Clarin, Ihor Kolesnyk, Stefaniia Kolesnyk, Yevheniia Marchuk, Anastasiia Markeliuk, Uliana Pasternak, Olena Pohonchenkova, Ruta Randmaa, Bohdana Serdiukova and Marharita Zavhorodnia. We also thank the translators: Yevhen Beliakov, Svitlana Bregman, Tetiana Fedorchuk, Yulia Kulish, Andrii Masliukh, Vitalii Pavliuk, Victor Pushkar, Mykhailo Tarapatov and Valentyna Korol.

Numerous people supported this project: Mireille Juchau, Olha Yaskevych, Yurko Prohasko, Ihor Kolesnyk, Roman Kechur, Oleksandr Filts, Bohdan Tykholoz, Oksana Kuzmenko, Luisa Passerini, Piotr Sitarski, Michał Pabiś-Orzeszyna, Natalia Otrishchenko, Natalia Aleksiun, Niels Brügger, Sara Day Thomson, Jeff Deutch, James Smithies, Paul Millar, Taras Nazaruk, Oleksandr Makhanets, Victoria Panas, Valentyna Shevchenko, Mariana Mazurak, Sofia Dyak, Iryna Sklokina, Beatrice Patsalides, Dagmar Brunow,

Billy Glew, Wojciech Owczarski, Ofer Dynes and Małgorzata Mazurek. Many thanks to Olha Stankevych for the research assistance.

We gratefully acknowledge the institutional and administrative support for this project from the Center for Urban History and Ukrainian Catholic University, both located in Lviv, Ukraine. Mykola Makhortykh from the University of Bern (the Institute of Communication and Media Studies, Switzerland) assisted with editing and translation of the diaries and helped to organize a series of online seminars where project participants could discuss the archival strategies of researchers in different areas of armed conflict. Katherine Younger, academic director of the program "Ukraine in European Dialogue" supported this project from the beginning and in 2022 diaries documenting received support from the Institute for Human Sciences (IWM, Institut für die Wissenschaften vom Menschen). The financial support for the project came from the 2022 Dean's Strategic Funding Scheme at the Faculty of Humanities and Social Sciences, University of Jyväskylä.

Finally, many thanks to Emilie Coin, Tori Sharpe, Yashika Tanwar and Khyati Sanger at Routledge for their unwavering support for this publication.

NOTES ON ACADEMIC
CONTRIBUTORS

Stephen Frosh has recently retired as a Professor of Psychology at Birkbeck, University of London. He has a background in academic and clinical psychology and was Consultant Clinical Psychologist and latterly Vice Dean at the Tavistock Clinic, London, throughout the 1990s. He is an Academic Associate of the British Psychoanalytical Society, a Founding Member of the Association of Psychosocial Studies, and an Honorary Member of the Institute of Group Analysis. He is the author of many books and papers on psychosocial studies and on psychoanalysis, from *The Politics of Psychoanalysis* (1987) to *Antisemitism and Racism: Ethical Challenges for Psychoanalysis* (2023). Other books include *Those Who Come After: Postmemory, Acknowledgement and Forgiveness* (2019), *Hauntings: Psychoanalysis and Ghostly Transmissions* (2013) and *Hate and the Jewish Science: Anti-Semitism, Nazism and Psychoanalysis* (2005).

Natalka Ilchyshyn studied psychology at Ivan Franko National University of Lviv. Currently, she is a Senior Lecturer at the Department of Psychology and Psychotherapy at the Ukrainian Catholic University. She is a practitioner with a specialization in family therapy, youth and children issues, trauma therapy. Ilchyshyn was part of multiple projects, such as "Trauma education and resilience project" (EMDR-Ukraine, 2022), "Core Skills in Emotionally Focused Therapy for Couples" (ICEEFT, Canada, 2020), "Trauma Psycho Social Support+" (TRAUMA AID Germany, 2021), and others. She was one of the three facilitators of the 'Two Months of War' project, and provided psychotherapeutic aid to participants: she gave students advice on how to maintain their anxieties and how to handle fear, and she also supervised group meetings.

Marguerite la Caze is an Associate Professor in philosophy at the University of Queensland, Australia. Her recent book publications include *Ethical Restoration after Communal Violence: The Grieving and the Unrepentant* (2018), and the edited collections *Hannah Arendt and the History of Thought* (2022), with Daniel Brennan, *Truth in Visual Media: Aesthetics, Ethics and Politics*, with Ted Nannicelli (2021), *Contemporary Perspectives on Vladimir Jankélévitch: On What Cannot be Touched*, with Magdalena Zolkos (2019) and *Phenomenology and Forgiveness* (2018). Her articles have appeared in venues such as *Contemporary Political Theory, Derrida Today, Hypatia, Philosophy and Social Criticism* and her current project concerns the portrayal of everyday resistance in film.

Chari Larsson is a Senior Lecturer in art history and theory at Queensland College of Art and Design, Griffith University. She holds a PhD in Art History from the University of Queensland. Chari's research focuses on theories of images, twentieth-century French intellectual history, and philosophies of representation. She is the author of *Didi-Huberman and the Image* (Manchester University Press, 2020) and has published in journals such as the *Journal of Art Historiography, Senses of Cinema* and *Psychoanalysis, Culture & Society*. Her current research project concentrates on the intersection of spectatorship, trauma, and the visual image.

Martta Heikkilä, PhD, is an Adjunct Professor and Researcher in aesthetics at the University of Helsinki. She lectures and publishes on the theory of contemporary art and aesthetics in the context of modern continental philosophy, particularly phenomenology and post-structuralism. Her current research project *The Work Beyond Aesthetics* concerns the concept of the work of art and its philosophical contexts during the past few decades. She is the author of *Deconstruction and the Work of Art: Visual Arts and Their Critique in Contemporary French Thought* (2021) and *At the Limits of Presentation: Coming-into-Presence and Its Aesthetic Relevance in Jean-Luc Nancy's Philosophy* (2008). Works she has contributed to include *Analysing Darkness and Light: Dystopias and Beyond* (2023), *Thinking* With – *Jean-Luc Nancy* (2023) and *End of the World* (2017).

Ihor Kolesnyk is an Associate Professor in philosophy at the Ivan Franko National University of Lviv. His recent edited collections publications include *Transhumanism: A New Paradigm for Humanity's Future; Contemplative Studies: Status and Prospects of the Scientific Field* (2022). His articles have appeared in venues such as *Visnyk of the Lviv University Philosophical Political Studies, Essays on Religious Studies, Gilea.,*

Philosophy and Social Criticism. His interests are oriented toward secular practices of meditation and their adaptation into higher education. He initiated a project 'Laboratory of Secular Meditation' to research different approaches to mind and its development.

Luisa Passerini is a Professor Emerita at the European University Institute, Florence, and was Principal Investigator of the European Research Council Project "Bodies Across Borders. Oral and Visual Memory in Europe and Beyond" 2013–2018. She has studied the subjects of social and cultural change: the African liberation movements; the movements of workers, students, and women in the twentieth century, and the mobility of migrants to and through Europe in the last decades. In this endeavour, she has used memory in its oral, written and visual forms. Among her books: *La quarta parte* (2023); *Performing Memory. Corporeality, Visuality, and Mobility after 1968* (co-edited with Dieter Reinisch, 2023); *Conversations on Visual Memory* (2018); *Women and Men in Love. European Identities in the Twentieth Century* (2012); *Memory and Utopia. The Primacy of Intersubjectivity* (2007); *Storie di donne e femministe* (1991); *Europe in Love, Love in Europe* (1999); *Autobiography of a Generation. Italy 1968* (1996); *Fascism in Popular Memory* (1987). With Tuuli Lähdesmäki, Sigrid Kaasik-Krogerus, and Iris van Huis, eds. *Dissonant Heritages and Memories in Contemporary Europe* (2019); with Gabriele Proglio and Milica Trakilovič, eds. *The Mobility of Memory across European Borders: Migrations and Diasporas in Europe and Beyond* (2020).

Magda Schmukalla is a Lecturer in psychosocial and psychoanalytic studies at the University of Essex (United Kingdom). Her research brings together critical theory, psychoanalysis, feminist/new materialist theory and art. She experiments with artistic, reflexive and ethnographic methods to construct psychosocial theories that can acknowledge sensual, repressed, fluid or unstable realities. Her work focuses particularly on the critical and epistemological potential of liminal experiences such as experiences of political transitions, migration, pregnancy and artistic production. She completed her doctoral studies under the supervision of Prof. Stephen Frosh in the Department of Psychosocial Studies at Birkbeck (London) and was awarded an ESRC Postdoctoral Research Fellowship to publish her monograph on post-communist experiences and contemporary art (*Communist Ghosts*, 2021, Palgrave).

Bohdan Shumylovych is an Associate Professor of Cultural Studies at the Ukrainian Catholic University and also works at the Center for Urban History in Lviv. He holds a doctoral degree from the European University Institute in Florence, a master's degree in modern history from Central

European University, and a diploma in art history from the Lviv Academy of Arts. His academic journey has been enriched by his participation in various international programs. Bohdan's primary area of expertise centers on media history in East Central Europe and the Soviet Union, media arts, visual studies, urban spatial practices, and the realm of urban creativity. His recent publication is *Soviet Media After 1968: Visuality, Corporeality and Identity.* (In Performing Memory: Corporeality, Visuality, and Mobility after 1968, New York/Oxford: Berghahn Books, 2023) deals with such issues. Bohdan is preparing a book about Soviet Ukrainian television and its influence on the social imaginary, to be published by the University of Toronto Press.

Magdalena Zolkos is an Associate Professor in the Department of Social Sciences and Philosophy at the University of Jyväskylä, Finland. She works in the area of political and cultural theory, politics of memory and affect studies. Her recent publications include *Restitution and the Politics of Repair: Tropes, Imaginaries, Theory* (Edinburgh University Press, 2020) and edited collections: *Contemporary Perspectives on Vladimir Jankélévitch: On What Cannot be Touched*, with Margeurite La Caze (Lexington Press, 2019) and *The Didi-Huberman Dictionary* (Edinburgh University Press, 2023).

CONTRIBUTIONS TO *DIARIES OF WAR AND LIFE*

Anastasiia B.	196
Iryna B.	90
Yelyzaveta B.	212
Olena C.	77
Oksana D.	94
Sofia D.	65
Mariana H.	207
Oksana H.	79
Anastasiia I.	233
Anastasiia K.	225
Anna K.	206
Dana K.	226
Ihor K.	68
Mariia K.	96
Miia K.	219
Oksana K.	224
Olha K.	43
Stefaniia K.	59
Kateryna L.	80
Anastasiia M.	64
Khrystia M.	50
Yevheniia M.	93
Daryna P.	245
Oleksandra P.	232

Kateryna R.   91
Ruta R.   73
Anna-Mariia S.   58
Bohdan S.   237
Polina S.   88
Sofia S.   72
Annamaria T.   244
Zhenia T.   54
Oksana V.   85
Viktoria Y.   83

IMAGES (1): DRAWINGS

6.1   Eva Alvor. (2022). Eskiz2   143
6.2   Eva Alvor. (2022). Eskiz6   143
6.3   Eva Alvor. (2022). Tryvoga   144
6.4   Anastasiia B. (2022)   144
6.5   Anastasiia B. (2022)   145
6.6   Anastasiia B. (2022)   146
6.7   Anastasiia B. (2022)   147
6.8   Anastasiia B. (2022)   148
6.9   Anastasiia B. (2022)   149
6.10 Anastasiia B. (2022)   150
6.11 Anastasiia B. (2022)   151
6.12 Anastasiia B. (2022)   152
6.13 Anastasiia B. (2022)   153
6.14 Ihor Kolesnyk. (2022)   154
6.15 Ihor Kolesnyk. (2022)   154
6.16 Ihor Kolesnyk. (2022)   155
6.17 Ihor Kolesnyk. (2022)   155
6.18 Ihor Kolesnyk. (2022)   156
6.19 Kateryna Luzganova. (2022)   157
6.20 Uliana Pasternak (2022)   158
6.21 Uliana Pasternak. (2022)   159
6.22 Marharita Zavhorodnia. (2022)   160
6.23 Marharita Zavhorodnia. (2022)   161

IMAGES (2): PHOTOGRAPHS

7.1   Stefaniia Kolesnyk. (March 07, 2022)   174
7.2   Ruta Randmaa. (March 10, 2022)   175
7.3   Ruta Randmaa. (April 16, 2022)   176
7.4   Anastasiia Markeliuk. (April 10, 2022)   177
7.5   Anastasiia Markeliuk. (April 10, 2022)   178
7.6   Anastasiia Markeliuk. (April 10, 2022)   179
7.7   Ihor Kolesnyk. (March 15, 2022)   180
7.8   Yevheniia Marchuk. (2022)   181
7.9   Ruta Randmaa. (March 10, 2022)   182
7.10 Bohdana Serdiukova. (May 13, 2022)   183
7.11 Bohdana Serdiukova. (May 13, 2022)   184
7.12 Bohdana Serdiukova. (May 13, 2022)   184
7.13 Bohdana Serdiukova. (May 13, 2022)   185
7.14 Bohdana Serdiukova. (May 13, 2022)   186
7.15 Lena Clarin. (May 13, 2022)   187
7.16 Olena Pohonchenkova. (March 10, 2022)   188
7.17 Olena Pohonchenkova. (March 10, 2022)   189
7.18 Olena Pohonchenkova. (March 10, 2022)   190
7.19 Olena Pohonchenkova. (March 10, 2022)   191
7.20 Olena Pohonchenkova. (March 10, 2022)   192
7.21 Olena Pohonchenkova. (March 10, 2022)   193
7.22 Bohdana Serdiukova. (February 20, 2022)   194
7.23 Bohdana Serdiukova. (February 23, 2022)   194
7.24 Bohdana Serdiukova. (February 24, 2022)   195
7.25 Bohdana Serdiukova. (February 24, 2022)   195

INTRODUCTION

Bohdan Shumylovych and Magdalena Zolkos

What are the psychosocial and cultural 'imprints' of war on people whom the war targets, affects and implicates, directly and indirectly? What is war for them as a *lived experience*? Attempts to address these questions necessarily extend beyond discourses of national security and defence, regional politics, accounts of the destruction to life, heritage and infrastructures, and the movement of people seeking protection from war, to also include categories and perspectives from studies of affect, feeling, memory, imagination, desire, creativity and the unconscious. They often combine registers of the extraordinary and of the quotidian in relation to 'war experience'.

This book addresses psychosocial and cultural effects of the full-scale war against Ukraine waged by Russia on February 24, 2022. It is a 'hybrid' book that includes excerpts of creative material (diaries, dream records, and images) and academic essays that offer analyses and theoretical reflections about that material. The creative material was created in Lviv in February–May 2022 as a project titled 'Two Months of War' in a joint collaboration of academics from Lviv Center for Urban History, Ukrainian Catholic University, and the Ivan Franko National University. It is a form of 'ego-documentation' (Dekker, 2002; see also conversation with Bohdan Shumylovych in this volume), intimate micro-historiography of violence (cf. Ginzburg, 1993), as well as a narrative and visual output of testimonial practices and of ethical witnessing (Felman & Laub, 1992; Oliver, 2001; Derrida, 2005). The material speaks closely to human vulnerability in the face of war and atrocity, casting into relief ruptures and ruinations brought about by the invasion. And yet, the material is also a collection of artistic and

DOI: 10.4324/9781003449096-1

poetic 'gestures of resistance' against violence, which occur through shared struggles, solidarity and endurance.

The project 'Two Months of War' involved production of narrative material, such as diaries and dream records, poems, photographs, drawings, voice recordings, and music (etc.) composed and created with a shared goal of documenting the cultural and psychosocial impact of the war as a lived experience. Around 60 students participated in the project under academic, creative and psychological mentorship, and over half of the participants produced written diaries, which became the basis for the subsequently organised, transcribed, digitised, and translated archive of war testimonies, titled *Diaries of War and Life*. The project combined embodied and experiential methodologies with creative arts and social analysis, as well as those of micro-history, feminist historiography and ego-documentation. Gradually, a thematic framework was developed by way of identifying shared motifs in the records, for example 'seeking shelter' or 'loss'.[1]

Accompanying the creative component of this book—excerpts from war diaries from the first months of the invasion—are ten academic essays and conversations, grouped into three thematic and conceptual sections. The first section reflects on philosophical, historiography and psychosocial aspects of recording lived experiences of war through personal narrativizations and images. Ihor Kolesnyk's 'Collective practice of meditation and phenomenology of consciousness in war' takes a point of departure in observations about instituting a 'safe space' in the 'Two Months of War' project that facilitated reflections, medications, narrativization of experiences and affects, and a communicative engagement with others. The key conceptual axis of the project, as Kolesnyk argues, was that of (preventing) a traumatic 'freezing' through application of practical methods and exercises that helped transform traumatic effects into creative and communicative practices. Drawing on the ideas of Harold Roth and the approaches developed within the Contemplative Studies Program, Kolesnyk articulates the theoretical category of a *subjective experience* of war as a psychosocial processing of the human encounter with violence and atrocity, and shows how it was developed at the level of creative practices of self-expression through meditative engagements, through 'critical subjectivity', through attunement to sensorial and affective responses, and through conversation and dialogue.

Following from that, Bohdan Shumylovych (in conversation with Magdalena Zolkos) reflects on the creative and historiographic output of the 'Two Months of War' project (*Diaries of War and Life*) by embracing the conceptual rubrics of ego-documentation and self-narration. Drawing on Michael Pickering's assertion (1997) that 'experience' is a central category of cultural analysis, Shumylovych elaborates the critical historiographic importance of war diaries (and dream records, etc.), discussing the multifarious ways in which they stitch together social perspectives with the inner life of the subject. The critical (and feminist) dimension of such narratives lies in the fact that they put out an array of traditional historiographic assumptions by insisting on the relevance of the everyday, and of intimacy, desire, and emotions, in depictions of war. As such, the documentation of the lived experience of the war is also a contribution to how the war is being inscribed in collective memory in Ukraine (and beyond). Finally, Shumylovych argues that beyond the psychosocial and historiographic records, these narratives and images of war are also political interventions, and he draws on Pasolini's figure of the 'firefly' to elucidate that dimension (see also Didi-Huberman, 2018)—these images and diaries appear 'in dark times' as expressions of resistance against violence.

Closing that section is an online conversation with Natalka Ilchyshyn (conducted by Bohdan Shumylovych and Magdalena Zolkos). This conversation raises the issue of mutism, or internal silence, which many Ukrainians went through at the beginning of the war. This is also one of the reasons why there are so few authors from Ukraine in this book, because local researchers could not guarantee that they would write a text due to the obvious circumstances. Natalka confirms the recognized fact that journaling or written self-reflection helps a person survive a period of uncertainty and that the positive or negative emotions we find in diaries show that experiencing an abnormal situation always has an effect on the individual. That is, we should remember that diaries were written by normal people who found themselves in an abnormal story. An important argument in this conversation is that it is not the reality or experience itself that creates trauma, but rather the individual's own socio-psychological reaction to wartime reality. This conversation also touched upon issues of guilt, shame, responsibility, and emotional instability. People who live (in Chari Larsson's words) a "quiet trauma" away from the battlefield are trying to work out their involvement in a common social body, but people on the edge of war have other tasks - they need to survive! It is important that both will have to learn to live together again when the war is over.

The second section, 'The Ruptures and Ruins of War', brings together academic essays that reflect on the different psychosocial and cultural impacts of war. Stephen Frosh in 'Dreaming of War' suggests that the diaries and dream records of *Diaries of War and Life* constitute a kind of 'dreamscape' of fear and desire. This is conspicuous in how these narratives convey the threat, turmoil and reality of war, in the evocative quality of what Frosh calls their 'emotional harmonics' and in their prescience. While the day diaries focus on recording 'actual events', there is a striking overlap between them and the dream records in relation to both the tone and content, and thus it makes sense to treat the diaries as extended dreams, and of the dreams as 'miniature diaries' that together narrativize anger, anxiety, and resilience. Deploying notions of brokenness and a phenomenology of grief, Frosh also draws on psychoanalytic ideas developed in previous European conflicts—notably those of death drive, melancholia, depressive anxiety and reparation—to examine how the psychosocial records of the 2022 invasion of Ukraine communicate the affective realities of war, as well as raise questions of justice and repair.

Next, in '"The Word Remains." War Diaries in Ruptured Time and Space', Magda Schmukalla asks how the pervasive sense that the war in Ukraine was not simply unlikely but *impossible* was shattered with the Russian forces' attack on Kyiv and other Ukrainian cities and territories, and to what cultural and psychosocial effects. The strikes on February 24, 2022, turned this 'unreal war' into a brutal reality, violently disrupting a sense of the self, of time and of the social order for those who were targeted and affected by it. Through her reading of the of the diary entries from the first months of the war, and by focusing on through-images, feelings and affects, Schmukalla examines these narratives in relation to psychoanalytic and psychosocial theories of rupture and asks how (and in which sites of social and psychic life) the disrupting forces of war were experienced and made sense of, and what feelings, thoughts and psychosocial matter was exposed due to these ruptures. Finally, she also explores whether and how war diaries become attempts at responding to (and resisting) a violent event that seeks to disrupt and dehumanise structures and life.

The next two chapters in that section focus primarily on the visual material from the archive. Martta Heikkilä explores the motifs of ruin and ruination in drawings and paintings, asking how ruins can be understood as traces of the war. In a theoretical sense put forward by Jacques Derrida, ruins mean that the viewer never grasps the image in the fullness of its meanings, but, rather, in facing an image they see its reverse—that which is invisible, the spectral absence that can be only caught indirectly by means of thought and memory. According to this deconstructionist notion, every image is structured by a loss; the image shows itself to us, but it never presents a totality of sense and thus remains, in Derrida's words, 'workless'. But ruins also have a more concrete sense in relation to the artworks produced in Ukraine in the wake of, and in response to, the February 24 invasion: through this visual material we discern some of the brutal force aimed at a physical and psychic devastation of a people. While the images attest to different dimensions of loss and mourning and to the destroyed security of life, Heikkilä's interpretative scheme also foregrounds a distinct sense of irony conspicuous in the images at hand.

In 'Quiet Trauma and the War in Ukraine' Chari Larsson investigates the relationship between trauma, vernacular photography and documentation of the everyday during war. The chapter starts with an observation that the photographic archive assembled at the Lviv Center for Urban History sits apart from familiar tropes of war photojournalism. Providing a powerful record of day-to-day existence that gives visual form to the disruption and dislocation experienced in the wake of the Russian invasion in 2022, these images yield new forms of visualisation of traumatic experience during war, which Larsson calls 'quiet trauma'. The 'quiet trauma' photographs are not filtered through the conventions of war photography; rather, Larsson argues they value lies in the capacity to attend to the civilian experience of war by those who might be located at a geographical distance from the direct armed conflict.

The third section of this volume, 'Resistance, Endurance, Testimony', brings into analysis of the material of war diaries theoretical perspectives from philosophy of emotions, cultural dream studies and affect theory to elicit these records performative force of building social solidarity, and of actively opposing and striving against the invasion, but also perhaps that of enduring the ordeal and the pain of the war experience. Marguerite La Caze argues in her chapter, 'Unexpected Shapes of Courage: Emotions of Resistance in Ukraine', that emotions can be expressions of opposition and defiance in the face of violence, as well as function as sources and inspirations for resistance. In a series of reflections on how the contributions to *Diaries of War and Life* articulate the emotional upheaval caused by the invasion, La Caze also draws attention to how their authors negotiated the effects experienced in relation to the disruption and horror of war. She identifies an array of emotions recorded in these diaries, including those that perhaps defy the conventional understanding of what living under conditions of war feels like (joy, love, gratitude and hope), while also noting the importance of anger, hatred and desire for revenge in the archival records. Drawing on the work of Marc Crépon on love and friendship as forms of refusal of violence and as counter-practices, La Caze interprets these emotions as signs of endurance, courage, and confidence and the will to survive, and the process of recording one's war experiences as an act of countering violence through care of the self and through communal solidarity.

In 'The Determination to Resist. *Dumky* by Young Ukrainians' Luisa Passerini approaches the diaries and dreams records as acts of resistance against war. She identifies in the texts alternating notes of doleful and cheerful notes, associates them with the work of Antonin Dvořák and the musical genre of *dumky*. The chapter starts with reflections on what creative interventions are enacted through acts of diary writing, including as interruption of the repetitiveness of quotidian life, as expression of courage and responsibility, as an act of risk-taking and as a process of subjectivation. Paying attention to the motifs of musicality and of embodiment in the diaries in the dream records, Passerini underscores their importance for memory formation, as well as explores their differential narrative framings (for example, in regard to the body, that of intimate haptics, reciprocal holding, protectiveness, precarity and vulnerability, etc.). In her analysis of dreams, Passerini notes that war blurs the distinction between the wake state and sleep, and connects them in wakes that allow for dreams to function as signals of hope and as manifestations of desire. As such, the chapter does not focus merely on the content of dreams, but reflects on the experience of reading their records—at a different time and space—as moments of connection, reciprocity and emerging solidarity.

The final chapter in the volume is 'Testimony, Endurance, *Tryvoga*: A History Open to Shivering Bodies' by Magdalena Zolkos, who, drawing on Georges Didi-Huberman's philosophy of representation, approaches the visual and narrative material of the diaries as depictions of political peoples. She argues that the diaries align closely with the notion of performative citizenship, which depicts social mobilisation and solidarity in Ukraine in the wake of Russia's invasion as an expression of the desire for freedom. However, in contrast to the dominant discussions, which privilege the notion of an active subject, the diaries depict the political people as irreducible to their deeds and undertakings, but that manifest also in moments of *withdrawal from action*—in the bomb shelter, in sleep, or during extended periods of waiting. A key corporeal figuration of these 'nocturnal peoples' in the diaries and images is that of shivering bodies, which Zolkos links to what she argues is a powerful affective motif in the diaries, *tryvoga* (a Slavic word signifying dread, anxiety, alertness, and trepidation). She concludes by noting the relational associations of *tryvoga* as endurance of a painful experience with others, and considers its implications for our understanding of witnessing war's violence.

The academic essays in this volume are interspersed with two sections that include excerpts from the diaries or other recorded testimonies (in English translation), created by thirty-three authors, and accompanied here by a selection of artwork images and photographs. The digital version of the whole collection (in the original Ukrainian and in English translation) is stored at the Urban Media Archive of the Center for Urban History (www.lvivcenter.org), which is a private institution based in Lviv, Ukraine, engaged in public history, research, and construction of alternative archives. For more than 15 years, visual collections (photos, amateur cinema, home movies, film news, etc.), oral historical evidence, and historical maps from the history of Central and Eastern Europe have been formed here. Since 2013, these collections have been combined into a single system of the Urban Media Archive (UMA). The archive's primary objectives encompass the collection, preservation, study, accessibility, and promotion of collections and materials often overlooked within the State Archives holdings. Thus, the focus of these collections is on private archives that show everyday life during the socialist era, unofficial or informal clusters of documents, or marginal collections that can often have the status of orphan archives.

The whole project is stored at UMA and is freely accessible upon registration (https://uma.lvivcenter.org/en/interviews, collection 'Two Months of War'). We hope that this digital collection on UMA can serve as a hub for the examination of historical data and the reevaluation of the broader role that archives play in society. This digital repository is dedicated to exploring and pioneering innovative methods for assessing, contextualising, showcasing, and applying diverse archival media and documents. It's important to note that the project is not focused on the development of tools for digitising archival materials. It is instead to foster collaboration among archivists, historians, and the general public, creating a cohesive community dedicated to the shared appreciation and utilisation of historical resources.

Georges Didi-Huberman astutely articulates that 'uprising is a gesture without end' (2016, p. 17), emphasising the enduring and timeless nature of the phenomenon of people rising up against oppression and injustice. The material collected, reprinted and analysed in this book shows that while resistance against war and violence can take many different forms, it also involves endurance and unqunechable desire for freedom. Invoking the figure of phasmid insects, Didi-Huberman (2016; 2018) underscores the point that uprisings, like gestures, are to be shared with others in the public domain, and he draws a parallel between the acts of disobedience, protest and resistance and the intermittent 'flashing light' of fireflies—both are signals of survival and non-capitulation. This poignant image signifies disseminating the transformative power of resistance far and wide. We aspire for the material included in this volume, creative and academic alike, to also signal radical solidarity with those who are actively engaged in resistance and in social transformation.

To read the online archive of **Two Months of War**, please visit the Urban Media Archive of the Center for Urban History (Lviv, Ukraine): https://uma. lvivcenter.org/en/collections/178/interviews

Note

1 Because of the sensitive and private contents of the diaries and dream records, we are not including their authors' full names.

References

Dekker, R. (Ed.) (2002). *Egodocuments and history: Autobiographical writing in its social context since the middle ages.* Hilversum Verloren.

Derrida, J. (2005). Poetics and politics of witnessing (O. Pasanen, Trans.). In T. Dutoit & O. Pasanen (Eds.), *Sovereignties in Question* (pp. 65–96). Fordham University Press.

Didi-Huberman, G. (2016). *Uprisings.* Gallimard.

Didi-Huberman, G. (2018). *Survival of the fireflies (L. S. Mitchell, Trans.).* University of Minnesota Press. (Original work published 2008)

Felman, S. & Laub, D. (1992). *Testimony. Crises of witnessing in literature, psychoanalysis, and history.* Routledge.

Ginzburg, C. (1993). Microhistory: Two or three things that I know about it. *Critical Inquiry, 20*(1), 10–35.

Oliver, K. (2001). *Witnessing: Beyond recognition.* University of Minnesota Press.

Pickering, M. (1997). *History, experience, and cultural studies.* St. Martin's Press.

PART I

Recording Lived Experiences of War through Diaries, Images and Dreams

1

COLLECTIVE PRACTICE OF MEDITATION AND PHENOMENOLOGY OF CONSCIOUSNESS IN WAR

Ihor Kolesnyk

Introduction: Context and Conditions

War produces very strong experiences. This is an opportunity to test common sense and the capabilities of the nervous system. Many Ukrainians and I would also like completely different experiences, ordinary human life with everyday challenges, but the reality is such that we cannot control all stories. War points out our vulnerability, helplessness, weakness, and inability of the mind to master the situation.

One of the glaring questions arises: is the mind capable of changing something in catastrophic history? Is the mind capable of not only describing, explaining, defining, and classifying but also helping people when undergoing a traumatic experience? How can we get out of this war with as few losses as possible, at least in regard to the mind, psyche, and body as frontlines?

In February 2022 we faced a situation when it was necessary to save ourselves, our relatives, and at least some kind of future. When we started the 'War Diaries' project at the Center of Urban History in Lviv, we tried not only to understand the events around us and not only to describe them, but also to create a special space of safety, where the participants would have a chance to find strength, words, and their own form of creativity. In my opinion, creativity is not only a means to switch from the 'anxiety'/'panic' mode, but also a method of transforming traumatic experiences into artefacts.

I will summarise the challenges and demands that the war posed to us in February 2022. It is with this baggage that we later moved into the project:

DOI: 10.4324/9781003449096-3

- a state of long-term danger to one's own life or the lives of the loved ones;
- complex emotions that arise in waves, depending on the situation at the front;
- the need to find one's own form of self-expression and coping with traumatic events;
- interaction with people in conditions where loneliness and alienation are only strengthened by the circumstances;
- the need for psychological support and return of confidence in one's own strength (mind, psyche, body).

The key goal of our *'War Diaries'* project, in my opinion, was to create a safe field where participants can apply meditative practices, achieve greater mental stability, become aware of their own inner experiences and thoughts, and find points of support in conversation with other participants. Over time, these experiences of traumatic events for all of us turned into creative artefacts: texts, recordings, poems, music, drawings, etc. Instead of freezing the trauma in memory 'until better times' to deal with in the future, we helped each other find our own healing rituals.

General Methodology: Phenomenology and Enactivism, Embodied Cognition, First-Person Experience

The ideas that we utilised in the project came from different academic disciplines, primarily from cognitive sciences, philosophy, psychology, and pedagogy, etc. Let's consider the main principles that partially formed the basis of the project's methodology.

In order to restore trust in personal experience, it was important to pay attention to the bodily dimensions of cognition. Our body and consciousness know the world through an inseparable perceptual unity, as elaborated in theories of embodied cognition and enactivism. We not only get to know the inner and outer world with the participation of our corporeality, but we also realise life's creativity in this system of coordinates: body–psyche–mind.

Paying attention to and putting trust in the body's physicality also helps with the sense of groundedness. While it is not a bunker or a reliable material shelter, it nevertheless forms a fundamental basis for a sense of security, a 'ground under the feet' for the mind. This approach is described by Evan Thompson in the introduction to the revised edition of *The Embodied Mind* (Varela et al., 2017, p.xxv):

The basic idea of the enactive approach is that the living body is a self-producing and self-maintaining system that enacts or brings forth relevance, and that cognitive processes belong to the relational domain of the living body coupled to its environment. One implication of this idea is that cognition requires the exercising of capacities for skillful action and that even abstract cognitive processes are grounded on the body's sensorimotor systems, including the brain systems that, as we would say today, emulate sensorimotor processes in an 'offline' way. Today, this idea of cognition as based on modal sensorimotor processes is central to the approach called 'grounded cognition', where 'grounded' means based on body states, situated action, and modal perception-action systems.

This approach to a certain extent helps with worldview (philosophical) challenges that arise in crisis conditions: the mind is feverishly looking for support, a new ontology, and a new epistemology. We need to affirm our own existence on a new basis (embodiment), to record in certain structures the internal experiences that arise in response to reality from the outside, and to bring them out in the form of knowledge. New pragmatic, personal experience-oriented ontology and epistemology need to be formed. What philosophers describe as a 'perspective of development' (Walach, 2014, p. 13), we were forced to produce at a fast pace due to the realities of war: '[i]n order to build a bridge, we have to transform subjective, inner experience into something that can be shared, i.e. subjectivity that is intersubjectivity. This is a first-person plural account' (Walach, 2014, p. 19).

We were not only forced to overcome the double taboo on subjectivity in scientific research (Wallace, 2000, p. 86)[1], but rather put personal experience at the centre of the process of a new ontology and epistemology. This new embodied, creative subjectivity, builds a bridge between living people and project participants in the process of live conversation, exchange of ideas, and sensory experiences. The format of our meetings included conversations in person or online, exchanging thoughts and feelings about the situation in which we found ourselves as a group. Eventually, we received results of this intersubjective interaction in the form of creative diaries, illustrations, poetry, music, and verbally expressed feelings. The experience of verbalized presence of others' own vulnerability was one of the most powerful aspects of our meetings. Paradoxically, even the lack of a 'scientific' method or formal language did not prevent us from opening up. As Harald Walach writes in 'Towards an epistemology of inner experience'

> The verbalization of the experience might be deficient. The experience might be too multifaceted to be able to be expressed in linear language. The emotional tone and the particular quality of the experience

will likely remain unspeakable, except, perhaps in poetry. (Walach, 2014, p. 19)

Creative expression naturally extended beyond poetry, and the partici-pants produced a significant number of artifacts in several expressive formats. All this became possible thanks to spontaneous reproduction of the conditions mentioned in contemplative psychology: conditions under which confidence in oneself, in one's abilities, and the right to express oneself, to be accepted in any state, is restored. In contemplative psychology, the emphasis is on personal experience and interaction with others. Private experience acquires its own objectivity and becomes the foundation for interaction with a much larger and chaotic world around. Our project was consistent with the goal of contemplative psychology, as elaborated by Han F. de Wit:

> [T]he aim of contemplative psychology is primarily 'first-person knowl-edge'; that is 'knowing' in the first-person sense of being wise, being free from confusion and ignorance [...]. It has a quality of intimacy and directness, and it is closely connected with being completely aware of one's life-experience on the spot. (de Wit, 2017, p. 417)

We also found ideas congruent with another area studies: contempla-tive studies. It combines the personal experience of contemplation (in various forms) with participation in the common experience of intersubjectivity, and with self-expression. It is also about translating these experiences and their results into the language of applied sciences (to build third-person knowledge), but this was not important for our project in its most active phase.

Our experiences during the joint project *'War Diaries'* resonate with ideas developed in the contemplative studies program of Harold Roth (Roth, 2006, p. 1795), where the key role is not only the abstract understanding of 'what is happening to us at the body/brain level?', but a direct understanding of a 'subjective' experience and trust in internal processes. We nurtured trust in personal experience through joint meditations thanks to 'critical subjec-tivity' and conversations (second-person experience, intersubjectivity), and left 'third-person experience' for later. Writing this text, I understand now that what we meant by 'for later' has finally arrived. The fact that I am still alive and able to write about past experiences of fundamental anxiety about life in the first months of the war is a testament to the great power of a vulnerable life.

Reading Harold Roth's texts now, I also realise that to a certain extent we, participants in the '*War Diaries*' project also managed to intuitively elucidate the importance of a living human exchange of ideas and experiences. The difference is that while we did that in the conditions of war, Roth implemented it in peaceful conditions of educational concentration:

> [T]he proposed concentration will emphasise the critical first-person study that is often found in the musical, dramatic, and visual arts and in laboratory science courses. By critical, we mean that students would be encouraged to engage directly with these techniques without prior commitment to their efficacy. They would then step back and appraise their experiences to gain a deeper appreciation of their meaning and significance. (Roth, 2006, p. 1789)

Another important element of our methodology in the project was contemplative practices, in particular several types of meditation practice. Usually, a much wider palette of techniques is applied to contemplative practices—from actual meditation to dance, rituals, singing, etc. In our circumstances, we had to limit ourselves to sitting practices, which I will talk about below (a full range of contemplative practices proposed for teaching in higher education can be found in the work of Louis Komjathy (2017)).

Meditative practices were also accompanied by phenomenological proce-dures of reduction and isolation of specific experiences from the chaotic flow of events. For us, it was important not just to dive into the depths of the psyche, but to practice the skills of 'swimming' in internal states and awareness. Contemplative studies by meditation aim to develop 'greater self-awareness, greater capacity to focus attention, and greater capacity to expand attention without losing precision or focus—in other words' (Burggraf, 2007, p. 1).

The foundation of contemplative phenomenological research is in a direct intimate connection with internal events, the consequences of explosions of informational and material 'things', like mines, bombs, and rockets (etc.). The applied meditation methods were aimed at achieving optimal states for transforming the energy of destructive emotions into something creative: instead of chaotic confusion, consciousness acquires a more 'stream' form as a result of practices (Thompson, 2006, p. 230). A relaxed and better-focused consciousness could finally find its way to creative expression (Barbezat & Bush, 2013, p. 9).

What Is Meditation and What Was Its Place in the Project?

Meditation is a concept used to denote a very wide range of practices in different contexts (religious, spiritual, secular, philosophical, scientific, etc.). When we talk about meditation, it is always worth 'prescribing' the coordinate system: (i) what kind of practices are these? (ii) What is their purpose? And (iii) to what context do they belong?

In our project, meditative practices were non-confessional methods of self-discovery from the first-person point of view. These practices are based on the principles of critical thinking, a phenomenological approach, and the values of respect, acceptance, care, and healing from trauma. The key function of meditation in the first months of the war was to stabilise the mind, the nervous system, and restore contact with the breath, body, and emotions. To a large extent, we tried to combine the phenomenology of personal experience and psychological elements of support in the process of traumatic experience. Regarding the psychological dimension of the project, the participation of Natalka Ilchyshyn and her experience of psychotherapeutic support in difficult situations played a big role.

In addition to stabilisation, the skills of trusting oneself, one's own mind, and its ability to adapt to incredibly difficult circumstances were important for us. As soon as we switched our attention from anxiety and fear for our own lives to internal processes that simply continued to happen autonomously (experiences, thoughts, breathing, sensory events in the body), the mind regained resilience to a certain extent.

In general, there are already quite a lot of descriptions of the application of meditation not only in scientific research but also in higher education. In contemplative studies and pedagogy (Burggraf, 2007, p. 2), meditative practices are used for educational purposes (to get acquainted with certain traditions or recontextualized forms). In psychotherapy, interventions such as Jon Kabat-Zinn's mindfulness-based stress reduction program (MBSR) are used to deal with stress. Scientists have investigated the impact of meditative practices on mental health and general well-being, which in some cases fits perfectly into the traditional context (Anālayo, 2019, p. 5).

The following dimensions of meditation were important for us: embodiment (Matko & Sedlmeier, 2019, p. 10), the ability to train attention and achieve closer contact with the observed phenomenon (Barbezat & Bush, 2013, p. 22), openness to experience and its acceptance. Over time, the experience gained could be translated into creativity and production of cultural artefacts.

The experience of meditation is always embodied—experiences are recorded in the coordinates of the breathing body, its parts, and processes. This is an opportunity to better understand yourself, your inner world, and also to find appropriate languages of self-expression and communication with other people. The story in an acceptable, intuitive form is a connecting link between my experience, the experience of another person, and other project participants. Meditative practices served us as 'intuitive pumps':

> Meditation, in the sense analogous to intuition pumps intended here, therefore, is a practice of performing mental state experiments in order to engender consciousness-altering, figure/ground frame-shifting, radical transformations of the philosophical gestalt of one's psyche, what I would call 'consciousness-raising pumps'. (Abelson, B., 2022, p. 65)

It also forms a link between us and those who will read, research, and experience similar events in the future. We are not only saving ourselves in this situation, but we are also to a certain extent saving (and shaping) our common future. The phenomenology of personal intimate experience allows us to know the manifestations of the external world, our internal reactions and, most importantly, to regain a vision of the structures that contain us, our self, integrated ontologically (through embodiment) and epistemologically (we can know and speak, manifest our own knowledge).

During our meetings in the project, we used secular meditation practices—without a religious context, prepared interpretations of experiences and integration them into ready-made abstract structures of knowledge. However, it is fair to note that certain ideas and techniques were borrowed from Buddhist traditions, in particular the matrix of questions based on the theory of perception (Anālayo, 2016, p. 1272), the principles of analytical meditation, and breathing practices. I discuss this experience below.

During the active phase of our project, meditation practices were used in several forms, including:

1 A 15-minute guided meditation session on March 6, which included a short introduction with attention to breathing and subsequent observation of sensations in different parts of the body.[2] If excessive tension was noticed, we let it go. Later, we added an element of visualisation and imagined a shelter, in which the participants had been previously. From the focus on imagination and memory we moved on to reactions in the body. We calmed down a little more in the body and later had a joint conversation about experiences.
2 A 15-minute guided meditation session on March 19, in which we first grounded ourselves through the sensation of breathing in certain areas, and later created a slightly more intense sensory field in the chest area with the help of hand placement.[3] Over time, we opened up to experience and listened 'to the heart', which could tell us about dreams, imagination, memories, feelings, and emotions (etc.).

3 A 15-minute guided meditation session on April 2.[4] We started with breathing, then we went through the parts of the body with attention, adding the rhythm of inhalation and exhalation. We paid attention to those parts of the body where muscle tension is usually concentrated (jaw, neck, shoulders, arms, stomach, chest, back, and legs). Finally, we talked about dreams.

4 Parallel to the project on April 30, I started the meditation course 'The Way Home', the recordings of which would later be used in various parts of Ukraine, including the occupied zones (Laboratory of Secular Meditation, 2022). Since the time for practice was limited in our sessions, I offered to engage in deeper experiences on the course whenever possible.

5 A brief talk about analytical, phenomenological methods of working with internal content on May 28. I put emphasis on questioning and on the 'non-verbal' nature of the cognitive process, especially in relation to the body, sensations, and emotions. This meeting was primarily about joint methods of psychology and philosophy for self-help and self-discovery. These were final instructions before the end of the active phase of the project.

6 A talk regarding instructions for working with our own music listening experiences on September 25. We created a music list in the first months of the project, which reflected an additional range of experiences of our participants (Музична мозаїка щоденникарів війни). Here I put more emphasis on the matrix of questions regarding the unfolding of phenomena in our perception.

Since the project was not exclusively focused on meditative practices, we used basic, intuitive skills and techniques. Breathing, body, tension, relaxation, acceptance of emotions, feelings, imagination, working with memories and dreams—the everyday experience of a person. In the conditions of the war, it was necessary to provide only the basis for closer observation, to form a kind of focus of experience, which later laid the foundation for the recovery of an individual from their traumatic experiences. I also wanted the trauma not to be 'frozen' in the future.

So, to sum up, in the project I applied the practices of mindful breathing, body mapping (scanning), visualisation, and analysis of perceptual experience based on emotions, feelings, visual images, dreams, and music. By asking ourselves the simplest questions ('what do I feel?', 'what is this feeling?', 'where exactly in the body?', 'what triggers these sensations and feelings in me?', 'where am I when I am aware of myself?') we helped the psyche and mind to find themselves and to prescribe basic coordinates. As soon as it was possible to do this, we observed for two months that it worked to a certain extent as the project participants slowly returned to routine and familiar patterns of behaviour. This was an indication to us that their mental state and reaction to events were slowly stabilising. Our 'War Diaries' slowly turned into a very intense archive of two-month records of *Diaries of War and Life,* narrated through various personal artefacts and collected in the cloud service.

Meditation and the transformation of trauma into creative artefacts: instead of conclusions

- The 'Two Months of War' project was our joint way, with the participants, to restore an environment where one could find a space of safety, one's own creativity, and through such creativity create a basis for further life. To do this, we first restored trust in our own minds and in personal experiences through various methods, and later we witnessed how creativity returned in various formats.
- The creative artefacts we have collected through our joint efforts attest to some degree that the project's goal has been achieved. If the mind is not stabilised, and the nervous system is agitated by anxiety and terror due to the threat of death, creativity does not find its way out. Diaries, dreams, stories, conversations, jokes, drawings, paintings, poetry, and music are evidence of courage, resilience, and adaptation to incredibly adverse and hostile conditions.
- As long as we are alive, our experiences are embodied. Accordingly, in the process of building a new ontology and epistemology in the conditions of war, it is necessary to take into account the body and its internal 'languages'. Trust in the personal inner world (subjectively) turns into mutual trust in life and enhances the ability to regain 'the ground under our feet' through lively conversations and interactions (intersubjectively). Under such conditions, the future finds some groundedness.
- The peculiarity of the project was that we did not conduct a social laboratory or experiment, but rather observed the emergence of various methods of support in 'field conditions'. The application of meditative practices has been part of my own experience for many years and was my contribution to the project. That which helps people to know themselves and to heal found a place in our meetings. I have great hope that the meditations have eased the difficulties of our shared history of war. I hope that the appearance of artefacts on the project testifies to a certain extent of living in a traumatic period without becoming 'frozen' in time, alienating part of the memory until the times when, supposedly, things 'will become better'.
- I must admit that the original motivation for participating in the project was not to write this chapter or to do academic research with subsequent

'serious' conclusions for academic readership. For me personally, this project became an opportunity to support others, to support myself, and to restore, to a certain extent, trust in the ability of the mind to think about the experience at hand; and thus, if not to change the world for the better, then at least to explain the madness around and to not let this madness destroy our personhood.

Notes

1 'In terms of scientific materialism, there is one taboo against scientific inquiry into subjective mental phenomena; and there is another taboo against allowing one's own subjective perspective to taint any scientific research. Thus, first-person, introspective inquiry into the mind is doubly taboo' (Wallace, 2000, p. 86).
2 Records of group meeting on March 6, *Diaries of War and Life*.
3 Records of group meeting on March 19, *Diaries of War and Life*.
4 Records of group meeting on April 2, *Diaries of War and Life*.

References

Abelson, B. (2022). Meditation and the paradox of self-consciousness. In R. Repetti (Ed.), *Routledge Handbook on the Philosophy of Meditation* (pp. 70–77). Routledge.

Anālayo, B. (2016). Early Buddhist mindfulness and memory, the body, and pain. *Mindfulness*, 7(6), 1271–1280. 10.1007/s12671-016-0573-1

Anālayo, B. (2019). Adding historical depth to definitions of mindfulness. *Current Opinion in Psychology*, 28, 11–14. 10.1016/j.copsyc.2018.09.013

Barbezat, D.P. & Bush, M. (2013). *Contemplative practices in higher education: Powerful methods to transform teaching and learning*. Jossey-Bass.

Burggraf, S. (2007, June). Contemplative modes of inquiry in liberal arts education. *Liberal Arts Online*. https://www.wabash.edu/news/docs/Jun07Contemplative Modes1.pdf

Komjathy, L. (2017). *Introducing contemplative studies*. Wiley-Blackwell.

Laboratory of Secular Meditation. (2022). *Шлях додому*. [Video] YouTube. https://www.youtube.com/watch?v=EU-cSkWs6g0&list=PLmtJwGxidHmN9cp Jxuy8s6DfV9brUtv3b

Matko, K. & Sedlmeier, P. (2019, October). What is meditation? Proposing an empirically derived classification system. *Frontiers in Psychology*, 10, Article 2276. 10.3389/fpsyg.2019.02276

Музична мозаїка щоденникарів війни (n.d.). [Video] YouTube. https://www. youtube.com/playlist?list=PL00cJOql59Gf63YDJrfNw274CmdK7YwpP

Roth, H. (2006). Contemplative studies: Prospects for a new field. *Teachers College Record*, 108, 1787–1815. 10.1111/j.1467-9620.2006.00762.x

Thompson, E. (2006). Neurophenomenology and contemplative experience. In P. Clayton & Z. Simpson (Eds.), *Oxford Handbook of Religion and Science* (pp. 226–235). Oxford University Press.

Varela, F.J., Rosch, E., & Thompson, E. (2017). *The embodied mind: Cognitive science and human experience*. MIT Press.

Walach, H. (2014). Towards an epistemology of inner experience. In S. Schmidt & H. Walach (Eds.), *Meditation – Neuroscientific Approaches and Philosophical Implications* (pp. 7–22). Springer International Publishing.

Wallace, B.A. (2000). *The taboo of subjectivity: Towards a new science of consciousness*. Oxford University Press.

Wit, H. (2017). On contemplative psychology, *Philosophy Study*, 7. 10.17265/ 2159-5313/2017.08.002.

2

'THE PRODUCTION OF FIREFLIES'

Searching for Truth and Truthfulness in the Diaries and Images of War, Conversation with Bohdan Shumylovych

Bohdan Shumylovych and Magdalena Zolkos

Magdalena Zolkos (MZ):	*Can you start by describing how the 'Two Months of War' project started? What motivated you and your colleagues, and what were your objectives?*
Bohdan Shumylovych (BS):	When Russia's great war against Ukraine began at the end of February 2022, I, like most of my friends, experienced a shock. Of course, we expected an attack, but somewhere inside we hoped that it was just a geopolitical game and that the Russians would soon withdraw their army from our borders. So the attack felt like something expectedly unexpected. The first few days we had to recover [from that shock], as we had no cash, it was hard to understand whether we needed to stock up on food, and people were leaving the city en masse. When my friends called me to join the regional defence unit, I realised that I had to evacuate my family from my city and took them to the mountains. This journey lasted 15 long hours, instead of the traditional three … everyone was running away … when I returned, the regional defence units [*ter-oborona*] were already filled with volunteers and there was no place for me, so I switched to another job I could do. There were refugees living in my apartment, at work we set up a shelter for people, and at the university where I teach, no one knew what to do in such difficult circumstances. And it was at that moment that I decided that I could help the students and wrote a letter to all the cultural studies courses (this is my program), suggesting that they collect war diaries. At first, a lot of

DOI: 10.4324/9781003449096-4

people volunteered, but later it turned out that many of them had what is known as mutism, they could not write and express their thoughts or feelings. An artist, Vlada Ralko admits: 'The first week of the war was numbing. Now I also have no words, except to call for the skies to be closed and for help with weapons. [...] Painting is my only language now. It's the only way I can say something for now. It's not even a weapon for me, but the ability to be alive' (in Hryshchenko, 2022).

MZ: *You say that the idea for the project originated, at least partly, in a desire to help and care for others (the students). Could you reflect on this ethical impulse - caring for others, feeling responsible to and for others - in what must have been a situation of a deep crisis and shock?*

BS: Human involvement during times of war is an intricate interplay of numerous psychological, emotional, cultural, and societal factors that stir individuals and communities to engage when the conflict emerges. The apprehension and anxiety caused by the onset of the war probably served as a catalyst for people to participate in various capacities, whether it entailed activism, volunteering, or even taking up arms for defence. At least this was what I saw in my city [Lviv]. In our media-saturated world, the exposure to the suffering and hardships endured by those affected by war elicits profound emotions of empathy and compassion. This frequently propels individuals into humanitarian endeavours, encompassing the provision of aid, support, or advocacy for those in dire need. Therefore, I think war [can have] a unifying effect on communities, whether they be workplaces or neighbourhoods. In the spring of 2022, I observed how people routinely came together to offer emotional, financial, and physical support to one another, strengthening their sense of belonging and active engagement.

As for feelings, all the experts I talked to emphasised that it was important not to introduce the project participants to introspection, but rather to help them reflect on what was happening around them. That's why we recommended describing how life in the neighbourhood was [affected by the war], changes to family life [etc.]. They could describe their daily routines, watch the media, and comment on events. We gathered the first group and decided to work in a scheme where the participants described their individual experiences, and at the end of the week, we gathered for a group discussion and looked for what was common in our experiences. We discussed words like 'home', 'house', 'hiding place', 'escape', 'refuge' … This way we were able to combine individual reflections and collective experiences. To make sure we didn't get into trouble in the group sessions, I invited Ihor Kolesnyk to the project, who is a philosopher specialising in secular meditation, and psychologist Natalka Ilchyshyn. Both of my colleagues taught students breathing exercises, we did various transference techniques, and talked about what to expect from our own bodies. This is how we lived together for the first two months of the war. We wrote, drew, talked about our war experiences … Later the administration announced that education at the university would resume and we noticed that fewer and fewer people were coming to meetings and writing diaries. It was time to let our group go, because it seemed to have done its job. I think for many people we worked as a secondary therapy and helped them cope with their own bodies in a time of chaos and uncertainty.

MZ: *You have used a striking phrase 'how we lived together' in the first months of the war. The relational dimension is very palpable in the diaries. While people's experiences obviously filtered through their own unique backgrounds, sensibilities, and subjective positions, there is also a strong sense of a kind of community forming and re-forming during these first months. Can you comment on this interplay of the singular and the communal in the project?*

BS: When we started the project, we realised that each individual would live this war in their own way, so we also believed that private diaries would become valuable ego documents. However, we deliberately invited the participants to communicate on a weekly basis to look for what was common in our experiences. In this way, we seemed to show that [for] each of us it was something singular, but together we created something new - a unique community. For many, this understanding was very therapeutic.

In terms of the national community - indeed, I have noticed huge changes happening among young Ukrainians; they realise their otherness from the influential imperial Russian culture, often switching between languages, quarrelling, suffering, and dreaming together. Ernest Renan once said that a nation is a community that 'suffered together' (1882/ 2018), for shared suffering unites more than joy does. He articulated the idea that periods of mourning hold greater significance in shaping a nation's collective memory compared to moments of triumph. This is because mourning periods impose responsibilities and necessitate a unified endeavour from the people.

MZ: *What response did you get from the students?*

BS: While we didn't actively solicit feedback at the time [of the project], reflecting on its impact with the benefit of hindsight, the participants said that it contributed to their self-awareness. It's essential to reiterate that our intention was not to steer them toward addressing personal fears, but rather to inspire them to capture a large narrative, to assume the role of historians chronicling the substantial and meaningful transformations they were actively involved in.

MZ: *And what were your thoughts and impressions when reading and viewing the material that the students produced in this project?*

BS: I can't say that I was separate from the collective psychosis that we were all experiencing. My family was living with a woman I didn't know in the mountains, I didn't sleep well, and I was on duty in various refugee shelters. I remember how one night a mother with two small children arrived, and I put them up for the night, but the mother was crying all the time. It turned out that her son, who had served in the army, died that day. I offered her to leave the children and return home to bury her son, but she refused. At that time, the train took ages to reach Zaporizhzhia (the family's native city) ... When I read my students' diaries, I recall stories like this as if their experiences are intertwined with my own and many other people.

MZ: *What were your main challenges and difficulties in the project?*

BS: The most challenging aspect of the project was maintaining group cohesion and diligently composing the daily diary entries myself. I distinctly recall feeling a sense of ennui when I penned my initial text back in the spring of 2022. To streamline the process and reduce the amount of writing, I adopted a practice of gathering images from social networks and archiving them online, resulting in an impressive collection of 500 images to date. However, the true struggle extended beyond merely existing; it was a formidable task to convey to others the profound significance of life itself and the importance of cherishing it.

MZ: *I am interested in the phrase you just used, 'the true struggle extended beyond merely existing'. I do not mean to undermine the enormous effort that people put into keeping their families, friends and themselves alive, but I also think it is worthwhile to reflect on the difference between 'surviving' and 'enduring' war, and how the diaries articulate that difference.*

BS: 'Enduring war' implies a more profound and long-lasting experience of conflict, suggesting that someone not only survives it, but also faces the challenges and hardships [the war] presents over an extended period of time. On the other hand, 'merely surviving' suggests a focus on basic survival without necessarily delving into the depth of the hardships and endurance involved. So, 'enduring war' emphasises the resilience and strength required to cope with the ongoing challenges of war, while 'merely surviving' suggests a more minimalistic view of making it through without highlighting the endurance aspect. In February 2022, I was reading a Ukrainian translation of Irvin Yalom's book, *Staring at the Sun* (2008), where the metaphor of contemplating the sun, which can destroy vision, means that one must look into death in order to appreciate life. Another metaphor that comes to my mind is that of Perseus and Medusa—a person who looks at the sun (death, Medusa) has a chance to die, so we need to come up with another way to look and not die. Perseus showed death to death, he came up with a way to survive. I think our project was a kind of a method - to look at death, but not to die, to come out of this test with dignity.

MZ: *And how did you cooperate with Natalka and with Ihor?*

BS: Natalka, a dedicated psychologist, had an extensive workload, tending to refugees, children, and individuals affected by the war who sought assistance in Lviv. Consequently, her availability for our group meetings was limited, especially when it became apparent that we were managing adequately and without major issues—during those times, her attendance waned. On the other hand, Igor was a constant presence throughout the project. His expertise in guiding us through breathwork practices was invaluable in initiating and concluding our sessions. Additionally, Igor and I engaged in profound reflections on the nature of embodiment, exploring how the human body interprets and internalises traumatic experiences. As a result, we embarked on a series of contemplative experiments, and now we are actively imparting our knowledge to students, helping them cultivate a deep 'embodied experience'.

MZ: *Let's move to more analytical and theoretical questions. Could you describe what kind of war archive* Diaries of War and Life *is? What is its cultural and historical value?*

BS: In the project's early stage, we successfully gathered 33 written diaries from students (out of a group comprising over 60 participants, though approximately half were unable to contribute written diaries). Additionally, we amassed a collection of drawings, audio files, reminiscences, testimonials, and dreams. We consider this collection as an important archive of various egodocuments of war. Historians commonly use the term 'egodocuments' to categorise autobiographical writings like memoirs, diaries, letters, and travel accounts. This designation was coined approximately in 1955 by

Jacques Presser, who defined egodocuments as texts where the author's 'I' is consistently present in the narrative, both as the writer and the subject being described. Presser played a significant role in publishing Anne Frank's diary and authored one of its earliest reviews. In his review, he emphasised not only the diary's significance, but also praised Anne's writing style (see Baggerman & Dekker, 2018). He acknowledged the challenge of setting precise boundaries for this term, suggesting that virtually anything could qualify as an egodocument. Citing musical compositions like Bedřich Smetana's 1876 string quartet 'From my Life' and Leoš Janáček's 1928 'Intimate Letters' as examples, Presser argued that the line between egodocuments and art was somewhat porous. In our archive there is a musical piece by Anna Kharchenko, whose parents still live in the occupied Energodar, a place of energy workers who service the nuclear power plant. It is a great egodocument of the war!

But historians still ask recurring questions: to what extent egodocuments, consciously or unconsciously, differ from the actual deeds and thoughts? How reliable is human memory or imagination, and how trustworthy are the authors? Presser alleged that egodocuments represented feelings and emotions connected to specific events: '[t]hey are conditions of vision, and spirit can see nothing not focused in some living eye' (Baggerman & Dekker, 2018, p. 96). Thus, the person's memory or imagination can never create a replication of the past, or a fair registration of life, since we know that people shape a fictive 'I' and from that personality, they assess life experiences, especially if this experience is heavily mediated.

The blurred boundary between historical egodocument and fiction is essential since a work of art could be treated as a form of imagination or creativity and at the same time as a diary and eyewitness of history. Presser observed that fictionalising in egodocuments is not a problem since both truth and truthfulness are important for history. When we deal with drawings, it is not easy to distinguish between 'truth' and 'truthfulness'. Images of war, like dreams, are important because they function as a reflection of real life; they include the conscious experience of life. An image holds a social dimension—it is shared, received, and interpreted in a particular manner. Its perception is intertwined with awareness and observation. Conversely, a dreamt image does not seek to be understood. Dreaming entails a sense of isolation, which, consequently, grants the dreamer a powerful gaze. Didi-Huberman stressed that paintings (or other fictional images) are, of course, not dreams: '[we] see them with open eyes, but this may be what hinders us and makes us miss something in them' (1990/2005, p. 156).

Reinhard Koselleck, while arguing about such recorded dreams as egodocuments, stated that historical reality takes its place from the split of two fundamental dimensions. The present is stored in the *space of experience,* both conscious and unconscious. Still, reality also intersects with a *horizon of expectation*, something that has not yet been experienced but which we can feel or desire (1979/2004, p. 255). Koselleck also argued that fiction or art is about possible and viable eventualities that control the imaginary. In this sense, experiences are like dreams, influencing us, even if we cannot clearly define them. The value of egodocuments is that they are the special source of the History unfolding before our eyes. Robert Harvey indicates that 'seeing clearly and effectively into the eye of history requires far more participation than just that of the direct witnesses' (2018, p. 92), because when people find themselves amidst war, whether near the battlefield or in exile, they encounter the initial moment of the Kantian sublime, evoked by the imminent threat to life.

MZ: *And what do you think about this archive as a contribution to the collective memory of the war that is currently taking shape?*
BS: I have a background in art history as my initial area of study. However, I later pursued a degree in history and completed my dissertation in that field. Interestingly, my passion for the history of art remains undiminished, and it has played a prominent role in shaping my career. Presently, I work as a public historian and hold a teaching position at the Department of Cultural Studies, a discipline notable for profound emphasis on the personal dimension of social interactions. In this academic field we delve deeply into how individuals experience and interpret specific social structures and arrangements. This approach illuminates the complex interplay between collective culture and personal inner experiences, offering insights into the potential transformations that can emerge within this dynamic. Experience, without a doubt, serves as a testament to the diverse manifestations of societal existence and plays a pivotal role in our daily interactions and connections. That is why we perceive egodocuments as material at the interstices of the private field and the social field. We also perceive dreams as social phenomena, and therefore for us it is important to collect them.

However, understanding the intricate mechanisms that underlie this relationship is far from straightforward. While we may attempt to draw boundaries between experiences rooted in specific contexts (like lived experiences of war) and those that are mediated (this is my personal experience of war), our lives seamlessly blend both dimensions. In contemporary times, the intertwining of localised and mediated experiences has evolved not only in scale but also in diversity. For a significant portion of the population, this fusion has steadily expanded over the past century, encompassing a wide range of experiences. Symbolic encounters are increasingly interwoven with sensory perceptions arising from our immediate sensory experiences, creating a rich tapestry of human existence.

The collective memory of this war is in the process of being created, and archives like ours help to articulate, imagine or even voice the embodied experiences of the war. We started with diaries since narratives play a pivotal role in how individuals derive meaning from their encounters and construe the societal landscape. Throughout our daily existence and within the realms of mainstream culture, we consistently immerse ourselves in various forms of storytelling. These narratives permeate our routines and shape our existence. They serve as social bonds, connecting us, and enabling us to reconcile the past and present in a meaningful way. According to Michael Pickering (2008, p. 6), experience holds the utmost importance in cultural examination as an intermediary concept that bridges the gap between modes of existence and methods of comprehension. The challenge of translating experience into language is a perpetual one (see e.g. César, 1992; Kruks, 2001; Jay, 2005; Caygill, 2020). Experience is not a static or predetermined classification but rather a dynamic facet of human beings that is subject to circumstance and variation. It navigates the spectrum between the known and the unknown, continually capturing the ongoing interplay between our identity and our understanding (Pickering, 2008, p. 29).

MZ: *Most of the authors of these diaries and images are women. Can you comment on the aspect of gendered subject positions and of feminism in relation to this archive?*

BS: Most of the participants in this project were girls and women, although two men led the group from start to finish. Ihor and I became the male voices of the project, which were minor in the crowd of female voices. One of the reasons why the project was dominated by women is that they were students of cultural studies, which is not considered a prestigious profession among men (at least in Ukraine). We can have from zero to three guys in a cohort of students, which is quite indicative of gender balance. In general, I think there are more women's voices in Ukrainian culture now, and this distinct change shows that our rather patriarchal society is changing. For many of the girls in this project, collecting diaries and creating records about life during the war was a gesture of resistance, and although they could not go to war, they 'fought' through their reflections and texts. It was their weapon, and I sincerely hope that among them, there will be those who will form the next 'voices', the voices of a new generation.

MZ: *And how about post-colonial perspectives?*

When I was a student in the 1990s, we never discussed colonialism or the post-colonial situation. We did not have academic courses on this topic, and there was no such discourse in general. Of course, we have traditionally heard the voices of political dissidents who, in the 1960s, turned to the works of Taras Shevchenko as the main anti-colonial poet of Ukraine. These voices declared our country to be a colony of the USSR, however, the post-Soviet situation was difficult to describe as post-colonial. I began to think about it more when I studied at a master's program in Budapest, and there were students from various countries of Eastern Europe, as well as Asia and Africa. But I took courses in imperial history in Florence, an educational institution where you could mostly meet students from countries that had once been empires. At that time, I had the feeling that colonialism or imperial history was more interested in those whose history is related to it, but I was not sure that students in Ukraine would want to take such academic courses. But now everything has changed.

Since the start of the Great War in 2022, the demand for colonial, imperial, or post-colonial studies has increased exponentially. Ukrainian intellectuals and artists constantly talk about the colonialism or imperialism of the Russians, suddenly, what was invisible manifested itself, and the poet Shevchenko once again became relevant for the young generation. Ukrainians are actively reading post-colonial theory and getting acquainted not only with authors from India but also from Africa and South America. The voices of people from the former USSR who critically look at the history of Russia and 'enslaved' populations are becoming relevant. But we still do not have an established discourse since Ukraine was also the founder of the USSR and also led a colonial policy in the past, of course as part of the empire (similar to Scotland, for instance). We fought in Afghanistan, and we still have monuments to the so-called 'Afghan soldiers', but there is little reflection that we were part of an imperial war. Parts of modern Ukraine were taken from our neighbours as a result of the imperial wars of the USSR, but we tend to perceive our geography uncritically, and our lands appear to be ours almost naturally. I say so much about this because I want to point out that we did not intend to introduce an imperial or colonial discourse into this project of writing diaries of war, but I think it is there. Colonialism is always also an individual experience, one that is constructed by social systems, and for those who have been colonised in one way or another, it is most difficult to find their own language, to understand 'who is speaking' and 'who is listening'. The war diaries project gives power over the language that describes the war—'they' don't do it for us, we do it ourselves, and in this gesture, there is strength and autonomy, and in this looking for our own 'language' (here I take it as a wide metaphor, more like discourse) there is also liberation from the colonial past.

MZ: *I am interested in this interplay between 'knowing' and 'not-knowing' in the diaries. This partly relates to what you said about the narratives not being retrospective, but a 'mapping' of the present. In this context, I wanted to ask you about the unconscious, especially (though not only) in dreams and fantasies reported by the participants.*

BS: One of the theoretical frameworks for collecting war testimonies and diaries is that individual stories may not necessarily be 'true', but their veracity and 'truthfulness' are also important for history. Here comes to mind the concept of 'intentionality' in phenomenology, which refers to the inherent feature of consciousness as directed toward objects, experiences, or phenomena. It signifies that every act of consciousness is not self-contained but rather characterised by its intentional relationship with something outside of itself. In essence, intentionality highlights the idea that our thoughts, perceptions, and experiences are always oriented toward or about something in the external or internal world. We grasp this external world on the level of invisible structures, which become embodied. This way, unconsciousness brings up reality but in a different way, like in a dream - it comes in the form of symbols or metaphors, images or stories that reflect invisible and embodied structures.

At a certain moment, students started reporting their dreams, and we also collected them. We considered such dreams not only personal but also social phenomena, which work with time. Cognitive neuroscientist Antti Revonsuo coined the concept/hypothesis of 'dreams as threat simulation', which suggests that one of the potential functions of dreaming is to simulate threatening or challenging situations. This idea aligns with various theories of dreaming, such as the threat rehearsal theory, which posits that dreams may serve as a kind of rehearsal for dealing with real-life threats or dangers. According to this hypothesis, during dreams, our minds create scenarios that involve various challenges, conflicts, or threats. These scenarios may be drawn from our real-life experiences, fears, or anxieties. By simulating these situations during dreams, our brains may be preparing us to respond effectively to similar challenges in waking life. In such dreams, people try to deal with time and reality in an unconscious mode.

MZ: *Following from that, I wanted to bring into the conversation an expression you used earlier in reference to the beginning of the war, 'expecting the unexpected'. One kind of dream that people had reported having before the full-scale invasion in February 2022 was what we might call 'proleptic' or even 'prophetic' dream; dreams about the war before it actually started. It seems to me that in these dreams people dare to think of something that, either in their own conscious lives or more broadly in the public debate, is unthinkable, unimaginable, perhaps even unbearable. Is that what you mean when you say that you, collectively, were 'expecting the unexpected'?*

BS: We held an online seminar about war dreams in the spring of 2023, and one of the participants told us that she had recorded people's dreams from before the war, and that they often featured bombings and enemy raids. Especially in the northern regions of the country, where a large wave of enemy attacks was coming from, people often dreamed of bombings. These dreams are also evidence that the constant information about the approach of the enemy equipment and military forces to the borders of Ukraine caused people to feel anxious (invisible structures?), and that this manifested itself in dreams. I personally had had [had seen] dreams a few days before the war started, and they were metaphorical about the war. So when I say that the war was unexpected, I mean that a full-scale invasion could have been foreseen, but that we had not wanted to believe it would. We expected it to happen and we did not expect it to happen, all at the same time.

I really like the metaphor of fireflies, which was borrowed from Pasolini. He noticed that in the 1960s fireflies disappeared from Italian nature and linked it to the image of capitalism and fascism, which kill individuality. The only chance to remain human is to shine in the darkness of uncertainty and chaos. Didi Huberman (2008/2018) talks less about capitalism and more about violence and images. I also love his thesis that fireflies are an image of hope and expectation. I think our project was a production of fireflies.

MZ: *Now I would like to ask you about the psychosocial dimension of the war. Do you think that the diaries and images give a unique insight into those dynamics?*

BS: I think that our project was not so much about uniqueness as it was about humanity. We, as a group of people, a certain community, attacked by the neo-imperial Russia, found ourselves in a situation of existential crisis. Even now, we are not sure whether we will survive in a state of such an endless war that aims to destroy our identity. But this horrible situation makes Ukrainians more sensitive and vulnerable to the misfortunes of others—now we often talk about the global South, about Africa, about conflicts that we had never talked about before. So, my insight is that we, as a community, are growing up, and maturing, to become more responsible for ourselves and others.

MZ: *You have used the phrase 'images of the self' in regard to the diaries and dreams. Can you explain what you mean by this phrase?*

BS: For this collection, I wanted to write a text about the relationship between visual and textual diaries created by my colleague, Ihor Kolesnyk. He has long been interested in the embodied perception of reality and practices of keeping visual sketchbooks. But I didn't have enough words, I felt some kind of constant resistance to the text. I wanted to describe in this text that for Ihor both writing and drawing are about the experience of himself at a certain moment in time, about the self that verifies reality. But what reality? Jean-Paul Sartre posited that reality is inherently subjective, moulded by individual consciousness and perception. He underscored the significance of personal subjectivity, freedom, and decision-making in forging one's own version of reality. Individuals enter the world devoid of a preordained nature or inherent quality, and they shape their identity through their decisions, deeds, and encounters. Put differently, individuals construct their own essence through the act of existing. Consciousness doesn't merely passively observe; it proactively interacts with and construes the world. Thus, Ihor's diaries are examples of existence, which articulates the 'self' and 'reality' through images and words. The wartime reality.

As humans, we may struggle to confront and comprehend horror directly, and therefore we rely on deflected or mediated images to make sense of it and to distance our own lives from it. This process involves transforming the horror into something imaginable, something that can be mediated through images and narratives. By using deflected images, whether through art, media, or other forms of representation, we create a buffer between ourselves and the raw reality of horror, and it allows us to approach and engage with the subject matter from a safer emotional distance. Therefore I see a certain value in the images produced during this project, since they are embedded experiences of wartime (they are real) plus buffers that help to distance the self from the real. The Lacanian 'real' maintains a profound connection to encounters involving trauma and intense emotions, encompassing both pleasure and pain. It comprises dimensions of experience that escape symbolic comprehension and hold the capacity to evoke deep emotional responses. Through the use of images, Ihor's diary constructs a framework that allows him to grapple with the horror of violence while maintaining a certain level of psychological and emotional stability. It is a way for him to confront the unfathomable without being overwhelmed by its immediate impact.

MZ: *One of the striking features of these diaries for me has been the frankness and courage with which their authors approach difficult issues and a kind of refusal to engage in idealisation, which can be very tempting especially when talking about a conflict where, as Jacqueline Rose puts it in* The Plague *(2023), the moral lines could not be clearer. Some examples of this frankness and courage are the account of uncomfortable or even 'unsuitable' feelings like being frustrated by and disconnected from when the dominant (idealised) image of Ukraine in the West has been that of unequivocal solidarity and unity. For me this is the true political moment in those diaries, the kind of dialectic between, on the one hand, people emerging as a collective in response to the war, and, on the other hand, the stubborn resistance against any notions homogeneity and unity, be it unity of feelings, of views, or of positions. The dominant characteristic of these diaries as representations of people is that of irreducible plurality.*

BS: I think that the value of this project lies in the fact that it was done by young people who will have to rebuild a war-torn country. And their feelings here are as honest as possible—they want it and don't want it at the same time, because responsibility is like growing up, it is both nerve-wracking and disturbing. Personally, I also have constant emotional swings and cry with joy when people collectively save someone (even the smallest cat) and hate them when they become infantile or aggressive. But these are all people; they cannot rid [themselves] of their humanity, and our project shows that behind the pose of official appeals, there is the everyday life of people.

MZ: *This brings me to the question of hope in these diaries and in the dreams …*

BS: Dreaming of peace is a powerful and positive aspiration. Many people around the world share the dream of living in a peaceful and harmonious society where conflicts are resolved through dialogue and [shared] understanding rather than violence. And I know that many people are dreaming of peace. However, in a recent survey of the Ukrainian population, the findings show a significant degree of confidence, particularly in the armed forces, a strong sense of solidarity, and optimistic hopes for fairness. People have an inherent sense of fairness and believe that individuals should be treated impartially and without discrimination. Injustice is often seen as a violation of this fundamental principle, and I think people at war or living through the war are dreaming about accountability. Justice holds individuals and institutions accountable for their actions. It ensures that those who harm others or engage in wrongdoing face consequences for their behaviour. I do not think we will have peace without justice, and such processes can facilitate reconciliation and healing, particularly in post-conflict or transitional justice situations.

References

Baggerman, A. & Dekker, R. (2018). Jacques Presser, egodocuments and the personal turn in historiography. *The European Journal of Life Writing*, 7, 90–110.

Caygill, H. (2020). *Walter Benjamin: The color of experience*. Routledge.

César, J. (1992). *Walter Benjamin on experience and history: Profane illumination*. Mellen Research University Press.

Didi-Huberman, G. (2005). *Confronting images. Questioning the ends of a certain history of art (J. Goodman, Trans.)*. The Pennsylvania State University Press. (Original work published 1990).

Didi-Huberman, G. (2018). *Survival of the fireflies (L. S. Mitchell, Trans.)*. University of Minnesota Press. (Original work published 2008).

Harvey, R. (2018). Eyes wide open: What the eye of history compels us to do. *Angelaki*, 23(4), 91–102.

Hryshchenko, I. (2022, March 11). Drawing is my only language: How Ukrainian artists depict war. *Birdinflight [blog]*. https://birdinflight.com/nathnennya-2/20220311-hudozhniki-zobrazhuyut-vijnu.html?fbclid=IwAR3AYcc572QJlzzcPDY8FtXy1mo-RJsyZL6btDWDTlNJ9M6UIJzShRy9eDU.

Jay, M. (2005). *Songs of experience: Modern American and European variations on a universal theme*. University of California Press.

Koselleck, R. (2004). *Futures past: On the semantics of historical time (K. Tribe, Trans.)*. Columbia University Press. (Original work published 1979).

Kruks, S. (2001). *Retrieving experience: Subjectivity and recognition in feminist politics*. Cornell University Press.

Pickering, M. (2008). *Research methods for cultural studies*. Edinburgh University Press.

Renan, E. (2018). What is a nation? (M. F. N. Giglioli, Trans.) In M. F. N. Giglioli (Ed.), *What is a nation? and other political writings* (pp. 247–263). Columbia University Press. (Original work published 1882).

Rose, J. (2023). *The plague*. Fitzcarraldo editions.

Yalom, I. (2008). *Staring at the sun. Being at peace with your own mortality*. Hachette Digital.

3

THE EMOTIONAL AND PSYCHOLOGICAL REGISTERS OF WAR

Conversation with Natalka Ilchyshyn

Bohdan Shumylovych, Magdalena Zolkos, and Natalka Ilchyshyn

Bohdan Shumylovych/ Magdalena Zolkos (BS/MZ):	*Tell us, please, how you have entered this project.*
Natalka Ilchyshyn (NI):	I joined this project at the invitation of Bohdan Shumylovych. The first day of war was supposed to be my usual working day. I had meetings with clients and work at the university scheduled. And at one point, everything stopped. Some part of me at that time needed to take care of my family and loved ones. To look for solutions that seemed best at the time. However, some part of me was trying to find a way to also 'extrapolate' this help, that is, to do my usual work. Of course, I tried to keep in touch with my students and clients. I provided counseling on psychological self-help in crisis situations. However, it felt insufficient. Participation in this project was my way of feeling useful in this strange time.
BS/MZ:	*Was your family with you at the time?*
NI:	Yes. My family and I—my husband and my three sons, aged 17, 12, and 7—we all stayed at home in Lviv. In Ukraine. It was our conscious choice. Of course, my husband and I had an agreement on how we would act in an emergency situation. Fortunately, we did not have to use this plan. We constantly received messages from our relatives and colleagues from abroad. Sometimes they sounded like

DOI: 10.4324/9781003449096-5

invitations. Sometimes they sounded like threats and accusations of inadequacy. However, staying in Ukraine and doing everything possible here, locally, was our shared decision and a manifestation of our life position.

BS/MZ: *Have you witnessed the effect of mutism, i.e. the inability to speak or write in the initial phase of the war?*

NI: Yes. I myself experienced a state of 'inner silence' for the first few days. I also noticed this in the participants of our project. It was very valuable for the participants to keep diaries in the way that was available and possible for them at the time, not only in the form of records and notes, but also in the form of art objects—drawings, collages, music, podcasts, etc.

BS/MZ: *What can researchers from other countries learn from the Ukrainian experience of war? Is there anything special you would like to tell us about collecting war testimonies and diaries?*

NI: The experience of war, of course, can be generalized, but it will always be unique to each of us. What seemed absolutely impossible yesterday may become your new reality at one moment. You can try to predict your reactions, 'train' certain skills and competencies, but it is also important to have compassion and acceptance of all your reactions, even the unpredictable and unexpected ones. Journaling and collecting testimonies can be a great tool for self-healing. It is important that this is done with the realization of absolute acceptance of one's own capabilities and inabilities, reactions, desires and abilities.

BS/MZ: *Did you use any special methodological approaches in your work with groups? Perhaps you developed some special approaches more appropriate in the context of war?*

NI: In this project, I acted as a person providing psychological support to the participants. I worked with the participants as a group of people experiencing collective traumatization. The focus was on understanding and acceptance of the processes that were happening to us and the participants at that time, developing self-help and self-regulation skills, reducing anxiety, and finding resources that could support us in these times.

BS/MZ: *What emotions do you think were significant, most prevalent, most strongly felt (by the participants of the diaries) in the first months of the war?*

NI: In the first days, weeks [and] months of the war, we experienced the entire spectrum of emotions and states—from shock, internal 'freezing', a sense of unreality of what was happening, to anxiety, fear, indignation, anger, hatred. At certain moments, it could also be euphoria and joy, and at others, shame, guilt, disappointment, a sense of hopelessness and meaninglessness of everything that was happening. However, we never tired of repeating to the participants of our project that all our reactions, whatever they may be, are normal reactions to abnormal circumstances. All our emotions are individual, and they all have the right to exist.

BS/MZ: *Can you comment on the fact that most (all?) of the diaries were authored by people who were not proximate to the combat zones? What is the psychological importance of this geographical and physical distance? It seems relevant especially in regard to the concept of trauma in that in its original psychoanalytic formulation, traumatic experience is thought to result from the immediate contact with, and proximity to, traumatogenic event. But these diaries give accounts of war trauma that does not involve direct exposure to combat or the experience of being a victim of atrocity.*

NI: Modern [theories] define psychotrauma as the experience of extreme stress as a result of events that a person perceives as a threat to his or her life, or [that they] witness. In other words, psychological trauma can be caused by both direct experience of a traumatic event or the experience of a witness to such an event, and by the knowledge of a traumatic event that happened to a family member or a person close to us. It is important to understand that it is not the event itself that traumatizes us, but the way we perceive it. If what is happening is too strong, unpredictable, or [too] long for us, it hurts us, regardless of how far away physically, geographically, temporally, or emotionally we are from the event at the moment. And this is very evident in our diaries. Of course, it is normal to take care of one's physical safety first, and many of our project participants sought such safety in other cities or countries. However, even at a distance from the immediate threat, the participants experienced these events as traumatic. Diaries, volunteering, and other forms of help and compassion could become a way for them to process their own reactions to these events, an opportunity to feel involved and regain a sense of empowerment. This is reflected in the diary entries. Instead, [and] this is my hypothesis, which obviously requires additional research, people who are in safe and close proximity to the combat zone have other priorities in life at that time—to survive.

BS/MZ: *What do you think about the role of sound in war's impact on the psyche and in how the experience of war is processed? The recurrent referencing of sounds and noises in these diaries is striking, as is their attention to silence. In these texts, the war registers through sound and noise, especially extremely loud sounds, but also more subtle audible events and phenomena. And, it seems, sound can have therapeutic and reparative dimensions, too, evidenced by the narrates of listening to music or hearing voices of loved that help achieve some calm and stability. What do you think about the importance of attending to sound and the audible in trying to understand how people experience war?*

NI: Most of us got our first experience of the war through sound. On February 24, I, like most of us, woke up to the sound of an air raid alarm. Then, gradually, other sounds were added to it—a lullaby sung by the mother of a fallen soldier during his farewell, the sounds of gunfire from military videos, and, finally, the echo of explosions in my hometown. Last year, when I was on a business trip in a safe country, I noticed that I reacted to any loud sounds, whether it was an ambulance siren or a tram. My body would tense up and react faster than my brain could analyze the source of the sound. Now and long afterwards, loud sounds will make us look around to make sure we are safe. Sound becomes a warning signal. However, music can and does become one of our pillars. When we discussed with the project participants the model of our BASIC Ph (a method developed by Israeli psychologist Mooli Lahad) [as one of the] resources, many of them pointed out how listening to music helped them cope, calm down, and reduce anxiety. At the moment when we receive the news of another rocket attack, it is so important for us to know that our loved ones are okay. When we call them and hear their voice on the phone, it encourages us [more] than any other [form of] reassurance.

BS/MZ: *A striking thing about these diaries is their psychic honesty, or frankness. They openly record thoughts and emotions that are seldom found in the more dominant discourses of the war, especially those found in many of its international representations, which frequently engage in idealization. For instance, the authors speak openly about being unwilling and afraid to participate in combat (contra idealized and stereotyped 'bravery'). Or they narrate resentful and negative feelings that people can have towards each other (contra representations of a 'harminious nation', of people unified in their shared struggle). There is no (or very little) self-censorship, disavowal and denial in the texts. Was that something you noticed in the interactions with the project participants, and how do you think about this aspect?*

NI: I agree with you. During the reflections at the meetings, we heard about very different reactions of the participants. In my opinion, this is a sign of a certain emotional 'maturation'. We have the courage to admit that we have different feelings and experiences—fear of taking up arms, irritation with loved ones with whom we have to learn to live together again, anger towards those who 'know better' how to fight and win …

BS/MZ: *Can you talk a bit about shame? It seems very prevalent and recurrent in these diaries. For example, people admit feeling ashamed for wanting to seek protection and safety in other countries, or because they are not putting more efforts in national defense, etc. Why would people who, objectively speaking, have the least reason to feel shame, experience it so strongly? It is others who, again, objectively speak, should be ashamed, the aggressors, or perhaps also those who are complicit with the aggression. Why does shame 'travel' the way it does; it seems to attach itself at times to the wrong subject, so to say …*

NI: Shame is a very powerful emotion associated with a moral imperative. The actions, words, [and] emotions [that cause] feelings of shame are determined by our value system, which was established in the process of upbringing and development, and by our own choices. In a moment of threat, when the need for safety and other basic things puts us in a dilemma, we can make different decisions. And if we feel an inner need to defend ourselves and our country, to get involved and help in any way possible, at some point we ask ourselves these difficult questions: Is what I am doing enough? Can I do more? Was my choice a worthy choice?

Can I still consider myself a Ukrainian if I am not in Ukraine now? How can I regain a sense of belonging? Obviously, the answers to these questions will vary. When I feel an internal dissonance between what is important to me and what is possible given the circumstances, I experience different emotions—shame, disgust, anger at myself, guilt. Our emotions are our reaction to what is happening inside and around us. But at the same time, they are a kind of 'marker' of our humanity and ability to empathize. I don't have an answer to the question of why the Russians don't feel shame, simply because I prefer not to think about them at all right now. However, I think the answer can be found somewhere [along] this plane.

BS/MZ: *Guilt is another strong emotion narrated in these diaries. It overlaps with shame, and yet it is also distinct from it. Is it important to distinguish between the feelings of guilt and feelings of shame in this context? What is that difference, according to you?*

NI: Yes, it is important. Feelings of guilt are usually associated with interactions with people or communities that are important to us. Guilt arises as a result of our awareness of the harm (real or perceived) caused by our actions or inactions. It is important to understand that no matter how 'external' the 'harm' may appear, it is always very real to the individual, as is the guilt that results from it.

BS/MZ: *One other recurring motif in these documents is fatigue and exhaustion. Is that something you noticed too, and how do you understand it? It is of course understandable that people are physically and mentally exhausted due to numerous factors, including the interruptions of sleep. Is exhaustion reported in these diaries a physical-mental condition, but also, perhaps, a symptom?*

NI: Yes, indeed, fatigue and exhaustion were noticeable in everyone—in the participants (this could be seen in the dynamics of creating the daily journals), in us, the people involved in organizing the project, and in everyone around us. Physical fatigue was combined with exhaustion of the nervous system. Undoubtedly, the lack of adequate sleep, the loss of a sense of security, and the possibility of restrictions in meeting basic needs [of] food, heating, etc., especially in the first days [and] weeks of the war, were taking their toll. However, the uncertainty about the further development of the situation, the constant flow of contradictory news, and horror stories from the occupied and then de-occupied territories [drained people's] emotional resources. It is a well-known fact that our nervous system is 'tuned' to temporary, [and] not long-term, mobilization. Stress [is] a way of coping with a difficult [and] threatening situation. Prolonged, constant stress without the possibility of recovery [and] relaxation very quickly leads to exhaustion and then to emotional burnout. The first weeks of the war were for all of us a 'time of held breath'. I don't know how clear this metaphor is? When we inhale, our body 'tightens up' as if to mobilize. When we exhale, it relaxes. Under normal circumstances, we take a full inhale and exhale. But in situations of tension or stress, we sometimes seem to 'forget' to breathe. Doubts, uncertainty, disturbing news, the need to make decisions, each of which could equally turn out to be both right and critical—all of this took away our emotional strength. However, the stage of exhaustion is also an element of the process of adaptation to new conditions [and] circumstances. Now, looking back, a year and a half after the outbreak of the war, I can say with gratitude: we succeeded! We held on!

Translated by Bohdan Shumylovych

EXCERPTS FROM *DIARIES OF WAR AND LIFE* (1)

Olha K.
February 24
Lviv, apartment at Pokhyla Street
7 am

vlad called and said the war started

February 26
Lviv, in a car to the Yaponska Street
i was sitting in the cellar of virmenska coffee house with a handsome man from Kyiv, an old teacher, and a family who showed me the way to the shelter. my hands were shaking, I took the alcohol from vlad, I left the keys to the neighbour. on Svobody avenue, I showed the way to the people in the street, got worried for what I just did, and they might turn to the wrong side, and I exhaled. A very young man in a military uniform and a little boy with a teddy-bear in his hands. i was so scared of that toy. then I saw Vanya from junior high. And Kholodnykh in Lev. It gave me a warm feeling.

March 01
Lviv, apartment on Yaponska Street

today is the beginning of spring. i can't help admiring people. i love everyone. everyone who writes about being alive, everyone who helps, everyone who does something, hugs, calms down, sends music, news, cooks to eat, strokes a cat, goes to the pharmacy, takes photos, or saves lives. what I thought to be my major burden is now my greatest advantage. I love people and i am grateful for having many of them around. ivan kostiuk is writing to

DOI: 10.4324/9781003449096-6

me, I'm asking for advice from sasha bul, mark nevil apologises for the harsh tone and asks foreign colleagues to trust Ukrainian photographers. we sleep on the floor, on the couch, in sleeping bags, very warm. it is very warm, although it is cold outside, we help and talk as if no misunderstandings ever happened before with the family from volhynia, with zhenia, with nazar. I love the sun but now I am afraid of windows. I do not know when I stop hearing sirens in my head.

i am very sorry to hear how some wonderful people scold themselves, as if they do not help enough. or, they feel ashamed that they are in a cosy place. me too, I was engulfed by this in the first days, and today I know that I am where i belong, in my city [...]

Today, we agreed with culturologists to write diaries of the war, and I began to reread what I wrote down the previous days and I do not know if I will be able to give it to anyone

March 02
Lviv, apartment on Yaponska Street

today is the first day since the beginning of the war when I cannot cope with my sadness. It has come up the first time in 7 days, before I only felt panic, joy, anger, and anxiety.

last night, I had my first panic attack in 7 days. in parallel, I was working on several difficult requests for accommodating displaced people and they got mixed up. while I was sorting them out, Tama offered to host a family with old grandmothers and children. A thought flashed through my mind to stop her from doing that because no one knew these people, and the bad experience of providing shelter to refugees on that day began to gain wide publicity through the word of mouth. The next thought was that if I made the previous assumption, I must have killed a human in myself, since they were old ladies and children. Immediately afterwards, I called another family who found it very difficult to find a place to stay all day because of the old-age granny who is hard of walking and can not use the stairs or sleep on the ground, and on the other side of the line I heard the dissatisfaction expressed about my offer. I went to take a smoke on the balcony, and the panic attack swept me. I recorded a voice message to Lis sharing that I it felt hard for me. I cried. my hands were shaking [very] hard. i could not write back to message requests. Then I recorded another voice message to some guy who asked if it was mandatory to register. i cried. another voice message to an acquaintance of mine about transfers from the railway station after curfew. i broke into tears again, and I was not able to stop for another voice message. the guys went out to the balcony for a smoke, and I could not stop crying and gasping for air. I felt so guilty that I could not pull myself together when people did not have time to calm me down. [...]

On the 24th, I woke up alone in an apartment at pokhyla str., among the under-packed staff half-ready for moving places, I was woken up by vlad's call at 7 a.m. he said I should immediately come and pick up the keys to the virmenska apartment, as he was leaving immediately, and that the war started. I would repeat several times that he his jokes were stupid, until I opened the news feed. I called my mother, while I was getting dressed, she started crying. for the last few months I have not been outside in the morning because the depression kept me in bed until the first working call. but even this experience made it clear that there were too many people outside as for 7:20 am. I went to check who was last time online on Telegram. do lis, marta, andriy know? i hesitate to call so early. I call myself stupid, because the war does not have the "early". marta and andriy did not answer. lis wrote that she was on her way to pokhyla str. I pass by an ATM where people are already queueing. that's right! I only have UAH 10 in cash for water from the vending machine. I hesitate whether to stay in the queue. while I'm thinking, it grows. I stay. I stand for 40 minutes, sirens go off. People are scared, hands are shaking, they are angry at the queue. no one dares to speak loudly, there's tension. then some man passing by, squatted to stroke a dog of a woman standing in line. it calmed me down. I take off 8 thousand – all I have on all the cards. they said the salary will be delayed. will there be any salary now at all? [...]

March 03
Yaponska

I sit in the kitchen in the dark, waiting for people from the railway station. Today, it was the first air raid alert that I slept through. 40 minutes ago, I didn't hear, neither sirens, no alerts.

My skin itches terribly, on my hands and my face. Maybe it's a cat allergy.

March 12
Yaponska

yesterday, vlad suggested going to france.

The siren woke me up today at 5 am (the alarm lasted for 2 hours).

We got along well with Dolka, she comes to me to get caressed. Tomorrow she will be taken to Poland. The first compulsive overeating for the war (cheese, cheese and pesto sandwiches, prosciuto, and chocolate)

March 13
Yaponska

Tonight, there were explosions near Lviv. Total devastation. I want nothing, I want to sleep, I would die to be able to sleep. The air raid alert lasted

3 hours at night. I couldn't make it and suggested going back to bed half an hour before the all clear signal. In the morning, I'm afraid of my night offer. It's like I'm sick of the whole world. I don't feel fear, even when I think about the death of my loved ones. My mother woke me up with tears in the phone call, someone told her that Lviv had been shelled. After that, Lis's mother wrote me a long message expressing fear for my life.

As shortly before as last night, everything felt as if life was back to normal. A full kitchen of guests, as if a couch-surfing family, as if our guests were not on a mission to film a war report, as if the Italian man that Danka brought along does not transport displaced people to the border. As if during the smoke break before going to bed they do not tell that their coordinators did not warn them to pack because Lviv may be the next target.

March 14
Yaponska

Today is a day of apathy and indifference. I have accepted the war and I guess, there is nothing I can do about it. Today, I attended a post-festive breakfast at marta's place, we discussed the family-type shelters they were working on. The discussion flew in an indifferent tone. while we were roaming around the bomb shelter in Franko Park, Sasha was telling how he saw a pile of dead bodies in Yavoriv. I don't care. I returned to the apartment that I started calling home (before that, the feeling of guilt did not allow me to) to find out that I was being evicted again. air alert started, I was hugging Andriy all the time while it was on and cried. Hopelessness, disbelief. I tried to search for options where to go next but there is no big difference between them. any place of stay can be destroyed, any apartment owners can show me the door; in any country, I [will] feel eternal sorrow and guilt. Vanya talks about the situation in Melitopol for an entire hour, I get tired of listening and getting shocked of the horrors. I want to sleep. I'm overeating again. While I'm washing my hair, I imagine a projectile smashing the bathroom and half of the house.

I don't see any dreams in my sleep but I often imagine bombs getting to where I stay and how they are tearing up my body. Sometimes I want it more than staying in the unknown, worrying, calling everyone I know, waking up from sirens and hoping for the best.

I'm tired of hating. Anger takes too much energy.

For the past few days, my stomach has been permanently sore and I feel like I'll never be able to fully wake up. I can't keep conversations going for long. I can't be friendly to the Germans.

March 15
Port, alarm went off

The first air raid alarm is far from any home, with potatoes and cola. The bartender closes the door, Vitalik asks if there was an air raid alert in the morning, or whether he was imagining things. [...]

March 20
Lviv, Fatset

It's scary to fall asleep
I do not take pills from Oleg
I am no longer late on my period.
I sleep alone, I saw a half-dream.
It feels anxious
I feel like I might die today.
I have stomachache and headache

March 21
Staroyevreyska, Lviv
01:48 am

It's been a long time since I've been out of bed because of the nighttime air raid alert. It might be because I am certain there are no important objects nearby. But now I'm sitting in the hallway, it doesn't make me feel any more comfortable. As the siren went off, I slid under the window on the bed, then an idea came to mind to go down to the shelter but I'm too afraid of the old stairs in this house. I put on my jacket, I'm sitting in the hallway, I've already imagined all the dangerous scenarios several times.
  I'm sick of it, I'm almost used to the war. [...]

* * *

The fifth air raid alert in a day. I'm sitting in Fatset. I tried to find distraction in work today but it is not enough to keep my focus. I think I'll find some other part-time [job]. I've never been so happy with the moonlight works that have finally reappeared. I write motivational texts, as notes to myself under the posts from the photos of Lviv. But I am incredibly tired. The Germans went home 3 days ago, before that we got drunk with the last beer they kept in the car. In the morning, the cars were evacuated. Today, their material was released in The Guardians. I read it and I felt disgusted to be there, among those words of war reporting. I don't know why, it's a very unpleasant feeling. [...]

The good news as of today is that Vlad's mom reached Lviv and we have accommodated her in the Virmenska place. The second good thing is the first mutual [love]. I never had mutual love, now I don't know for sure if I got it. This is also a certain self-rescue instinct. Not staying alone—being with someone, redirecting attention and caring. Whatever it is, it worked all the time while I was living at Andriy's place. Yesterday was the first night of the war that I spent by myself and it was creepy. My half-sleep turned into sleep paralysis and the worst thoughts that had taken all my power until morning. […]

March 26
Notes in the phone, Lviv

Yesterday, a dad of Vika from DK was killed in the front. Here we go. The acquaintances are leaving. Today, it's a dust storm in Lviv. The wind blows you off your feet.

4:28 pm
air raid alert while in the waiting line for tire fitting near the southern moll. […]

March 27
Yaponska

Recent weeks have been just bad. I can't distinguish between triggers, shades; I just feel horrible all the time. […]

I can't find the strength to work well, to read [and] study texts, or just fiction, to read anything that is not a news feed for the day. I have no power to respond to friends from abroad or elsewhere. I'm just really tired.

Yesterday, I wanted to be a suicide murderer. I'd like to rush in somewhere with a bomb and blow up as many enemies as possible. I have no energy to live but dying just like that, without taking a single Muscovite with you, seems somehow stupid.

Stupid low pressure, I keep feeling nauseous, I feel dizzy and my fingers go numb. And I can't feel like complaining because of it, because whimpering […] about low pressure during the war still does not seem appropriate, although I have already made an appointment for a manicure without thinking that it might not be the right time.

* * *

'Explosions open up the heart', Stas said today as he explained his [uplifted] mood. And then we were standing there, silently [looking] at the blue, blue sky in the Lev's courtyard. […]

April, 1
Yaponska

Today, like several previous days before, I feel very bad. Low blood pressure or fatigue—who knows. My mom and my brother arrived for several hours, we had a 15-minute meeting. I can't remember the last time I was so happy to see my mom, we have never had [a] close and warm relationship.

I keep having more episodes of overeating, hours of stupor, when I can neither work nor rest. However, I can listen to music again and sing along [...]. But most of the time, I feel like my whole body is going to get numb, or I'll blink my eyes and never wake up again. It's like I have permanent nausea for everything that happens and comes to mind.

April 03
i'm viewing photos from Butcha.

i am silent all the smoke break on the balcony with Andriy. I am thinking about how to get russian citizenship, and on the day when no one is expecting I would arrange the biggest terror attack in moscow. I want their wounds to fester forever, so that they drown in a viscous thick swamp, choke in agony, burn alive in fire, can never fall asleep, lose their minds from fear, get scared of every sound, so that their children would go grey-haired, die of hunger, so that they would lose loved ones in front of their eyes. I want to be in every Ukrainian soldier who strikes the last blow at the occupiers. I want to stand near every russian mother who would perpetually unfold a bag with the remains of her son. I want to be the darkest darkness that persecutes them and catches them. I want to cut every apolitical person with a blunt knife. I want to give away everything I have, my life, my home, only to take away more from them. My desire for revenge will stay with until the end. I have no other dreams. I will never forget it I will never forgive it. [...]

some few hours ago we had a meeting of illustrators where we had to create the anti-stress book when you can destroy pages with all things russian. at the end of the meeting, the idea was raised that aggression does not solve anything and that it is all too much. I agreed with that because I would not be happy from that as a user. we decided that we should focus on something more good.

and now I feel like not carving the appliqués from a booklet, but their living families.

i hate it.

Translated by Svitlana Bregman

Khrystia M.

March 01
Kalush

I lived every minute of this day. I felt like a molecule, an element of a huge atom. I think every Ukrainian was the same today. I already knew that the school sirens should have sounded in Lviv the day before, but I did not expect to hear them today at eight in the morning. Using the logical-deductive method, I guess that if yesterday the siren was educational, then today it is real. No one can confirm or deny anything yet. I put on a dressing gown, opened the window, and realised I wasn't dreaming: the siren sounded under the very house. I went out into the corridor, where the panic started even before I woke up. In the corridor, Maria was clearly panicking, her eyes were foggy. I asked something, but in response saw frightened eyes and packed bags: everyone was running to the basement. I didn't not believe there was a need for this, called Vasylyna, and heard her voice, "Girls, this was [a drill]. And in general, I am now at the liturgy, join me if you wish'. That's it. I told the girls that it was [a drill]. They didn't believe [it]. I entered the room, and in a minute the girls behind the door calmed down and said, "Ah, it was [a drill]." At that moment, I could not yet realize that a full-scale war had begun in Ukraine. Russia suddenly invaded our country and began bombing airports and military units. What do I know about war? Will the books I once read, the movies I once watched be useful to me? [...]

The most nervous phase began when I was deciding how to get my sister [Sofia] to leave Kyiv. It turned out that Russia attacked at five o'clock in the morning and fighting and explosions in Ukraine had been going on for at least five hours. Many people, either thanks to intuition or intelligence, had already left – some were on the road, and that caused long traffic jams. I found out that there were no tickets, there was no blablakar, hitchhiking was unreliable, there were no seats, it was scary, the trains were delayed, and there were some rumours that the trains were no longer running. I couldn't keep calm at the liturgy, being distracted by a phone call with Sofia. My mother and my aunt Lena were calling in tears … The first few minutes were indescribable.

I'm standing near the church. [...] Next to me is a ten-year-old girl with a backpack and a bag in her hands. Her mother is staring at one point as if she is looking for someone, waiting. The girl sways with her bag. She asks her mother, 'I just want to be sure. Mom, call dad, please. I just want to be sure'. In response, the mother continues to look at a far, far point on the horizon and refuses with incomprehensible sounds. This woman is in a panic. It is difficult to even find words at such a moment, especially the words to say to a child. A minute later, the girl says to her mother again,

'I just want to be sure. Where is dad? Shouldn't he be here already? Mom, why is it so difficult for you to answer? I just want to be sure'. I want to intervene, look into her eyes, and say that dad will come, and everything will be fine, but I don't know if I have the right to do so, a moral right to tell lies.

March 02
Kalush

Today I decided these notes would be like a job. I am trying to catch history. I am healing myself and trying to describe the common feelings of all Ukrainians. Yesterday I was in despair.

I am writing now from the bomb shelter. The situation is tense. For some reason, there were two sirens in a row. It is rare for Kalush. It's strange. Am I afraid? I'm afraid now. There's a heavy lump in my throat, like a stone. I can't move. I can't speak. Everyone near me in the bomb shelter is discussing the news. In Kyiv, a rocket just hit the area of the underground passage at the train station1F613 I'm afraid. I am afraid that these words … I do not believe these words will be the last. But if … If so, I don't know. I want to cry. I feel cold all over my body. I'm afraid. Who to shout now??? Everyone is in the bomb shelter. [...]

I'm writing now and trying to capture everything because I don't know WHAT tomorrow will bring. I really don't know now. Just yesterday I fell asleep knowing that I could sleep enough, seven hours. Today I am not so sure. I love life. No matter how ridiculous and desperate it sounds now: I just love to live, I loved it before that. I fell in love with life even more when I started studying at the university and met incredible friends and sisters in spirit. They know who I'm talking about! Now I shudder at every sound and look around the room searching for my backpack and bag. As our Kharkiv guests (not refugees, this is a stigma) say: you don't need much to survive, literally one backpack is enough, but to LIVE, to live in comfort, you need much more.

I really want to sleep, but I can't. You need to hold on and stay awake, because today can be difficult. I feel like I am fighting on every possible front, so I take a part in this war! I feel how it affects me. I go volunteering with the sincerest thoughts. I don't have a hint of pathos or hypocrisy. I do it because I can't help it. I believe. I believe in the Ukrainian people. [...]

March 04

[...] Every sound paralyses me. As soon as I hear something like a siren, I stop breathing so that not to overhear it. My heart instantly starts beating fast, I jump up and open the window. Siren. I know I have only two bags I take down to that basement. I also take [my] two cats. It's like a game. Everyone runs to the basement with a backpack. [...]

March 05
Kalush

[...] There is silence now. Silence in the city. The anxiety and tension have subsided, and for the second night, I sleep in more or less usual clothes for sleeping. Such silence gives me time to recover: to take a shower, to rest as much as possible in the conditions of war, but at the same time, I feel alert. [...]

March 07

[...] It hurts to realise that the war will not end soon. The news about the family from Irpin [that] was [evacuating] from the city simply made me speechless. It hurts me so much, it's so hard to realise that a whole family, a whole family of four with small children, died! Died when they fled the city with their suitcases. They died while they were running away so as not to die ... How can that be! How can this be allowed now? But so as not to fall into apathy and despair, I do not allow myself to concentrate on this for a long time. On losses. This is a defensive war, and losses will take place. Unfortunately, this is a very bitter truth. By the way, Arestovych says that those who are away from hostilities, for some reason, experience more pain, cry more, suffer more ... I am ashamed of this. What moral right do I have? All my relatives are safe. Me too.

March 08

[...] [A] dream I had was about Vlad Nimak, my friend, who is now volunteering in Kharkiv. Some kind of high-rise building, Nimal is filming everything below from a great height. Later, he jumps from this high-rise building with [.] belay, but the belay, which for some reason is around his neck, looks like a white ribbon. Nimak jumps swinging in different directions. He doesn't seem to be suffocating. I don't know what's next. [...]

March 09
Kalush

Two hours before going to bed, I was reading the news until my brain simply said, 'drop the phone'. I don't want to write anything. There is nothing to write. There is nothing to write about ... ? Where are my emotions? Today we 'walked' with the people from Sumy. I'm not a talker, I feel desperate. I'm slow. I just go with the flow and do what everyone else does. I read the news, ban Russian channels, make emotional videos and posts, I volunteer, and I rarely take a shower. [...] I made a video for the Russians, and at the end, I wanted to ask them to do something, but not to protest, because it didn't work very well. I asked Yarem, and he advised me to ask Russians to commit suicide. Joke of the day. The events in Mariupol shocked me to the bone: they bombed a maternity hospital, and a children's hospital. People, due to constant shelling, cannot be buried properly, so they are thrown into mass graves ... Russia will regret this for years. It will never be pardoned. This is sacrilege. This is madness. This is hatred of people.

March 12
Border

I am on the road to the place where Kristof, a friend of my godmother, with whom we spontaneously left Ukraine, will pick us up. Why? Why do I do that? I still don't know. I don't know why I left. Going there, I felt like I was in a fever: should I go back? The people on the border are so kind that I feel uncomfortable because I was not harmed in any way, I saw no shelling, my house is undamaged, and my city is not bombarded. It is I who must stand there at the border and help everyone. A nice guy, with whom I spoke English, helped us with things and transport. If I don't find a place to be useful for Ukraine, I will literally go back. But I hope I will find it. [...]

This war will last long. This war will not be over in a month. Even two. It's all just beginning. I can't believe it. I don't want to believe it. I refuse to believe it. But I will have to believe it. I am going to some village in the south of Germany, and I know I will stay there for more than one month. I have never been so uncertain about things. [...] I will never be the same again. I feel all the unnecessary shells fall behind me, and something substantial remains, not for long, but remains. I grasp it, and then it hides somewhere again. I grow a rough layer of impenetrable skin. This little thing is very vulnerable. Let's put it this way: I'm very vulnerable when it comes down to it, and that's when I feel absolute honesty with myself, absolute devotion, and purity. [...]

March 15
Place: doesn't matter, some village

I finally found the answer to WHY I still went to Germany, if it was quite calm, quite safe in Kalush. I volunteered, and studied medicine, why did I go then? Did someone shoot me in the back? No. But the first days I walked around like a nervous, electrified hedgehog and ruined the psyche of my mother and younger sister. I used to half-open the window for the first ten days so as not to miss the siren. I [kept] myself awake so as not to miss the siren. I used to set an alarm clock for every hour at night and usually missed it all the time. [...] I was a walking bomb that could explode at any time. [...]

Translated by Genyk Bieliakov

Zhenia T.
February 24
1:03 pm

I'm ashamed to acknowledge it, but I've been waiting for this war for the last couple of months. Apparently, every generation has to live through their own trash: my great-grandparents have survived the Holodomor and World War 2, my grandparents knew the Soviet Union machine, and my parents saw its grandiose collapse. And what about me? I had this thought that even "Maidan" is "not mine."

I wished for this war to happen because I thought it wouldn't affect me, as "I'm_in_Lviv." I would just look at it from beyond my window, not even leaving my apartment. But it would be real, pulsating. One would be able to touch it. […] And here I am, sitting on a mattress in the hallway, as it's safer here, realising that I don't want any more of this war, I don't want to say that my generation has survived it. […]

March 02
Evening

I'm devastated by the news and constant help requests in chats. I'm angry at war. It irritates me. I want to shout "Enough!" to the "Nexta" channel and the channel of Verkhovna Rada with their endless news reports, even the good ones. The only message I want to see now is "russia has capitulated."

I'm exhausted from constant air alarms. […]

March 04
12:48am

I can no longer stand the war. It's the second time when I dream of myself and my friend drinking at Kolos, and I literally drink one beer after another, and the time in a dream is the same as in real life.

I went to a coffee shop today, and I was so ashamed of myself.

The war never lets you go, never lets you forget about it. […]

It's excruciating to hear about people dying and people who might yet die, about the ruined cities, wrapped and dismantled sculptures in the Lviv city centre, about people saying they won't ever come back here under any circumstances, to realise the pause the russians have put our life on. It's also scary to see the enemy and not react properly, freeze, or get afraid. It's scary to appear as an absolutely different person once/if they come here. What's also scary, is that it will still be painful once the war is over. This horror breathes in my back, but when I turn around, I can't see anybody behind me. […]

March 14
4:40 pm

[Yesterday] I learned how to use the assault rifle. [...] The next day I went to my parents to pick up my grandfather's air gun to train the posture and movements. I think I'm doing better now. I wrapped it in an old sheet and took it to my place. [...] Once you have at least minimal control over the situation (you can seal the wound, shoot an assault rifle, start a car), you feel calmer. I hope I won't need these skills.

March 15
10:30 pm

I noticed two interesting things within these 20 days [...]. First, distance. Its perception has changed a lot with the advance of enemy troops and their terror. I remember the horror when they started assaulting Kyiv. Before February 24th, I'd thought that if there was a war, it would be somewhere in the East or next to the border towns, that they wouldn't be able to advance further (I hadn't thought that the war is waged not only on the ground but in the air as well). And here you go, Kyiv, 5 hours away from Lviv by IC-train. But when the orcs started attacking the Western cities, Kyiv faded away, and I was very worried about Frankivsk and Lutsk. Both are around two hours away from where I am. The next stage came after the Yavoriv military base strike. It's 30 or 20 km from Lviv. The war crept in, and I had to realise that my safe zone was no longer 600 km, it was 20 km. Later, I went outside and realised that there was a military hospital right in front of me. Yavoriv military base stopped being that scary after this realisation. My "it's so far yet" went through a hundred transformations during the war. Now, I'm not thinking in terms of finding a safe city in a war-torn country, but rather in terms of finding a safe place in a war-torn city.

   Second, the relevance of news or conversations. Never before have events unfolded so rapidly. In the past, I rarely read any news or analytical texts about politics. [...] Before, we could discuss the events for weeks. Today, we discussed particular news for two hours max. The situation is constantly changing, and decisions are made one after another. For me, these 20 days of being in the information field feel like 20 years, and it's not an exaggeration. As if the world and our country live in a 2x mode.

March 22
10:00 pm

It turns out that hatred can be very sweet, intoxicating, like strong mulled wine. There is a chat where there is a military man of the UAF and a Russian woman. The former texted about the dead bodies of the russians lying around him. When I imagined the russian woman reading it, it was so funny that I laughed to tears. I started imagining those bodies, the way they look, the way they return home in the bags. All these little details amused me, I wanted to know the tiniest details (don't tell me that it's immoral or "too much"—there is no "too much" when it comes to the occupiers). Hatred used to tire me. Today, it ignited me, it gave me strange energy. This is the hatred that makes you laugh—loudly and frantically.

April 05

I remember this feeling of stability and solid ground very well. One doesn't have to distract oneself from bad thoughts, one doesn't have to recover from anything. I remember the exact day when this solid ground started fading away. It was the end of September. My boyfriend and I went to our friends' birthday party at Keiserwald. There, I was told that our old acquaintance fell under the train and was in a coma. It's as if something was taken away from me.

The end of November. My wonderful grandpa received a CT scan—50% of the lung damage. Covid takes him away and me with him. I become fragile and vulnerable, somehow tiny. Ever since, when I didn't work or study, I turned on [the TV] in the background. I learned to mentally repeat the hero's phrases to not allow myself to think at all. I fell asleep with a podcast on. It had to play all night, as the night was the worst. Sleeping pills, cigarettes, lots of food, and lots of cheerful light series to be able to flee at least there. It was February, I had just gotten used to life without him, and that's when the war started. And it started again: series 24/7, food, cigarettes, podcasts. Today, I watched the last episode of the series, and I was really worried—what now? Today, my life is all about forgetting and remembering. Painful remembering: my grandpa and the war, two strong blows, forever.

I remember the time when I wasn't afraid to remain silent and think for a couple of hours very well. The time when one doesn't have to flee to the imaginary better worlds. I used to have my own one. Now, my world is inferior, shaky, dark, and bizarre—it's like an empty city after the bombing.

April 22
01:49am
Polish-Ukrainian border

I went abroad for a while. To Portugal through Poland. I had to return a forcefully displaced cat to her owner. [At the last moment] I realised that the new carrier was 6 cm bigger than allowed. I thought it was the end. I thought I'd have to invent a story about the cat fleeing the explosions and having no time to take the carrier. Honestly, I was really worried about it. But then I drove to the checkpoint and saw the eyes of the border guards: they looked at me, scared and slightly sympathetic, so that I wouldn't think that they were making a victim out of me or that they were too careless. They were very cautious with their questions and their looks, they could only guess what the person staying in front of them went through—maybe, she didn't see a war, but maybe, it took away all she ever had. No unnecessary questions able to touch on a sensitive topic, almost no questions at all. They only asked me if my cat had a chip, and when I said that it had and started looking for a passport, they told me they believed my word. Something tells me that it's a general attitude to Ukrainians among the foreigners. They keep a sympathetic silence lacking the right words.

Translated by Vitalii Pavliuk

Anna-Mariia S.
Before the war

I remember in the last weeks before the war I had very vivid dreams, all like full-length bright films. In these dreams, I always travelled, woke up in another country, city, circumstances ... I saw a lot of familiar faces, it seemed as if I remembered everyone I saw at least once in my life. I will not retell every dream, but I dreamed that I was at the funeral, I dreamed that I was in the hospital, I dreamed that I flew to America without documents and things, just got on the wrong place and was not even asked about the ticket, and then I had a dream that I was running away from bullets, as if in Hollywood blockbusters and put in a kennel to escape. It was the last such vivid dream and it was somewhere after February 12, when thoughts of war were in my head. [...] Everyone has been talking about the war since the end of 2021 as if Putin will definitely attack at the beginning of 2022. [...] I didn't want to believe [it], I didn't want to talk about it and nobody knew anything for sure. [...]

Translated by Victor Pushkar

Stefaniia K.
February 24

Today we woke up earlier than we would like to. The accompaniment was beautiful – an air raid alert. [...] Fear will cripple you more than [any] war. [...]

I'm calling Stefko. I listen to how he says that he terribly loves me, a bunch of soothing and encouraging words. [...] In the background, the girls talk to their friends. They're crying. I'm about to break down into hysterics, too, but I promised my mom I wouldn't panic.

[...] I'm rushing to pack that wretched grab bag but I don't even have a backpack or a bag. There is only a suitcase, but nothing will fit in there. And I don't even have a normal jacket here. Why would I? People can't be prepared for [war]. Someone tweeted the poem like that. Ohhhh ... I am helplessly looking around my huge pile of belongings.

[...] It hurts so much that we have to go through this. That Ivan and Ira have to experience this. That we all have to experience this. Why can't this bloody stolen scrap-work parody of a state just fuck off?

We joined the online class. We were sitting there and crying. What are you left with? There's nothing you can do about it, stay there and be afraid.

February 25

[The air attack alerts] turned me into an animal scared of the night-time. Now, the shadow in the sky entails the shadow in the brain. I calm myself aggressively, I disengage myself, I write from time to time. I turn my head to the window: how peaceful and beautiful it all looks. And it could be another Friday night and I'd be lazy surfing YouTube. It hurts me the most. That everything could be fine, that I could just enjoy life now, and never bother. It hurts to tears and I feel like beating someone up. [...]

March 04

[...] I saw sirens in my dream. I was in Korosten, outside, with Ivan (my brother, 9 years old) – we were fishing from the ice-hole in the puddle in our yard.

Suddenly, there came the [...] familiar siren wailing, I pulled his hand to the hallway, and then I thought maybe I wasn't even dreaming about it. I opened my eyes – but no, it was a dream, indeed.

Somebody is screaming. It got to realise that through dropping into the dark. The screams came from the street. It was far away, but strong. I'm sure that's how people with a ripped limb would scream. It was a man's voice. [...]

March 06

It was impossible to wake up, I barely opened my eyes at 13.20. For the first time, I didn't sleep in jeans. Blissful bliss of the blissful bliss. Morning news scrolling is demoralising because I find out that my Korosten and the neighbourhood is being [hit] hard. Fuck. [...]

March 07

Why am I falling into so many dreams? Why can't I wake up at all? Did my body decide to wait for all this in an anabiosis? The body is so heavy and sleepy, as if fogged up, the neck hurts as hell. And this has been many days now. [...]

You just have to exhale, you can't panic. I can't control what happens there, I can't turn back the rockets with my bare hands, I can't. Ex-haaaiii-liiing. Shush, shush, shush. Now, at the moment, everyone is alive and safe-and-sound, and that is the main thing.

The girls want to hug me and soothe me. I'm grateful to them, really, very much. But this [does not] work with me. I can't hand over my suffering to someone. [...]

March 08

[...] Mom called, she said: "Is it possible to buy bandages in pharmacies over there, in general? If there are some, get me as much as you can, I will send you the money, and you send it to us by Nova Poshta delivery service (!)." Well, it would not seem so weird if [she] didn't work in the hospital. When the hospital has no bandages, you need to tackle things on a larger-scale.

Well, I'd love to, except I'm not good at all these operations. Actually, I am here as the very same intellectual front (yeah, and what would you think). Well, it's good that now everyone you know would volunteer somewhere, and every other acquaintance volunteers with humanitarian supplies. I am writing to Stefko

I'll try to figure something out.

Bandages are available

We can send them

I immediately cheered up, but I still had to find some transport. Should I forward it by train to the district center? Should I send it by mail? I get on *KorostenToday* (don't ask) and see that there is the heaven-sent Anatoly, to my delight, who will go tomorrow from Lviv to Korosten by minivan and will be able to pass on anyone/anything. I delegate the arrangement with him to my mom *smiley of a stupid moon*1F31A My mother drops me an even longer list. Holy cow, it's really bad in their hospital, what do they even have there at all?? I'm starting to get nervous for the safety of all the people of Radovel *twitching my fingers in anxiety.*

We managed to find almost all items on the list, we made arrangements with Anatoly, packed the box, and I'm so happy. [...]

March 11

I catch myself thinking that I feel relieved when running down the stairs to the bomb shelter. Well, we couldn't expect not to have the alarm signals any more. The legs are shaking, the head is spinning – the bastards woke me up at 4:44, they pulled me out from a deep sleep.

We dragged our feet back and dropped off to sleep. I am warming up under two blankets, falling into oblivion. I reluctantly look out, with a huge effort, check my phone – there's an air raid alert again. And here we tango back again to the bomb shelter.

Now I am morally and technically going to make an effort and go out on a medication procurement trip, and also to get some necessities. If it doesn't work, I'll delegate it to the humanitarian staff.

There's nothing in the brain right now. That's how fatigue feels. What am I tired of? Because what did I run into today or from life in general?

March 12

[...] AIAIAI. I WANT TO SLEEP, GIVE ME A KNIFE, I'LL CUT OUT ALL THE ruZZians, AND THEN I'LL FALL ASLEEP. [...]

March 22

[My family] came all together, to see off Ira, Ivan and Grandma Liuda leaving for Poland. It was spontaneous and unplanned.

I was so happy to see them all. As if everything was really good and they just came to Lviv to celebrate my birthday together. [...] We settled legal issues, repacked their bags, sent the dupes to the bus station, and put them in the car. We exhaled. That's it, three of them are now safe.

My parents and I went to have some ice cream in Stryisky park. We had a nice walk and talk. They treated me to some delicious meals, told me a bunch of all the good things, kissed, gave me some money. [...]

March 25

When we are awakened by the quiet dawn,
we will hear the sun rise
on a new day the earth is tired, it is thirsty after winter,
it will resurrect, it will warm up,
the white keys will open the sky and we will be out of the habit

and scared to look up
and someone's voice will flow like a river to melt
and twist
The paths will lead home all, the living and the dead, and the weary
and the candle of remembrance will burn.
in pure hearts, bare and exposed

April 04

[...] My Godmother writes on Insta that it makes sense to indulge into not reading the news. Because the role of observer or eye-witness is also traumatising. She's a cognitive therapist. Must be true. Butcha.
BUTCHA. [...]

April 05

I don't remember what I saw in my dream but it had the sirens. And I would wake up from time to time to see if I was dreaming or not.

I feel like my fear went down. The initial panic has disappeared. It's like it's completely dissolved. I can feel the ocean all around me. So quiet, with ripples on the water surface. But it was so HEAVY. Like a warm and weighty blanket. Or, is it the other way around: am I the ocean? Am I in the middle of the ocean?

Not important. The point is, there's pressure and weight all around. And it's not unpleasant. It's just there. You can live amidst it all.

Today's dream resembles something very ragged, three times twisted, and in several dimensions simultaneously.

Because we were woken up by a siren at 5:30 am. What a shame, because I slept so well. Here's what, kids, this is why we ripped out their tongues and fingernails. [...]

I'm so unnaturally tired – I am just a body.

April 06

I had a dream about my son again. First time in a very long period. But, I'm sorry, that's not the way to start. I don't have kids, I haven't any, and I hope I never will. It's just that every now and then I dream that I have a son. I have become accustomed to him in my dreams, as well as to a baggy dark silhouette who sometimes chase me down the stairs, along the asphalt and labyrinths.

My boy and I were in the occupied Korosten. A bunch of Z letters, a decimated ATB. People must undergo checks all the time. They checked on me, too. They ask: Do you know that the war has been going on for two years now?

Two years? And I thought that it was 12! – I reply in either an ironic manner, or I'm lying. I listen to a bunch of "liberating" bullshit and I drag the little one behind me, through the rubble. [...]

April 18
Today it's not us.

In the morning, at 7:44 am, the air raid alert went off. We went down, as usual. Pajamas, battered, sleepy. In general, we were calm. We've been sitting there for forty minutes. The girls are sleeping, Maria is clicking something on the tablet. I can hear some movements – a woman rushes in, short of breath: "May I come in here!?". Kozlovsky puts her on a chair. A woman begins to get hysterical, she says she doesn't want things, she cries. I'm irritated and snuggle into Gelia's orange blanket. Creating a panic, it pisses me off. Now, there a bit more people in here: those who usually ignore the sirens have joined today.

There are no deaf ears in the shelter – there's someone saying that they saw a rocket from the window, the woman continues to howl "there explosions are so terrible." It's a good thing we can't hear anything, I guess.

With somebody whimpering in the background, and with wehaveseen themissilefromthewindow-itwassobig-therewassomuchsmoke, I felt the abominable creepy shiver in my stomach. The one that used to live in my guts in the first week. I escaped from it into my cell phone. We bake pizza, we develop business, we exhaust our eyes. [...]

Translated by Svitlana Bregman

Anastasiia M.
April 09
(*From a dream diary*)

I was at home. Then my friends and I decided to go camping. I didn't know our purpose, but it wasn't just for fun. They said we would be able to cross the Dnipro River at a ford. These people were from Western Ukraine and used to the shallow Carpathian rivers. But the Dnipro is a very deep river; one can't wade across it. I also recalled that they dug an artificial canal in the middle of the Dnipro to deepen the riverbed. Moreover, I can't swim. So I was going to certain death. I wanted to tell my friends about it, but I couldn't. I was ashamed of it. I thought: "Okay, I trust them". We waded across a small creek and headed for the Dnipro. Then everything ended. Next thing I know, we go somewhere as if along Sivash. Salt and black mud are all around. We go. I don't see those people anymore. I see my mom and someone else I can't identify. We go. We reach the destination point. It turns out to be a kids' camp. It is underground. We go 2 or 3 floors down. Everything seems very strange. They give us a tour. It has some patriotic orientation. But why is it underground??? This question does not stop worrying me. Everything looks very gloomy and scary. If I were a child, I would go crazy there. It doesn't seem like any fun there. The place is empty. Apparently, it's off-season. We pass through the rooms. It's a very strange maze. I would get lost if I was alone. Then we go outside. I ask my mom why we came here. She says that this is her alma mater and there is no need to be afraid. She used to be in this camp too; it is very old. She used to be a strong woman and her nickname was Horseshoe. It's all very strange ... Then we go home. We come to the church I went to when I was a kid. It feels like Easter is coming. But people are already commemorating the dead. I can't understand whether it's a church or a cemetery. Everything is mysterious. There is a crucifix to the right of the temple door. Mom wants to go there. I guess she wants to kneel at it. But there are two women. They are my classmate's mother and her sister. They are very hostile. I ask my mother not to go there. I want to warn her about the danger, but I can't because this feeling of danger seems illogical. I have no proof for it, so I keep quiet. She goes there. It turns out that instead of a crucifix, there is a stove, and she is going to cook us dinner. I ask my mom to go home. But she is really going to cook. Those women make fun of her, but she doesn't understand it. I am very sad. I stay and wait for her. I feel irritated. I want to go home, but I can't leave her.

Translated by Svitlana Bregman

Sofia D.
February 11
(From a dream diary)

At night I also dreamed, I don't remember exactly, but I remember that there were a lot of … in short, I was standing somewhere and there was one mouse and a lot of little mice. But the little mice are so small, like, you know, newly-born kangaroos, they were just running around like fleas … like some bugs, in general. There were so many of them, and they were running around. And at first, I was afraid that I would step on them because I really stepped on one, you know, it was someone's mouse, not just a conditional rat. It was someone's mouse, someone else was standing next to me trying to calm me down. And then there were so many of them that I started to panic, I started to run away from them. I felt like they were crawling over me, so I started to shake them off, to walk around, and all that. And then I was woken up by the siren.

March 03
8th day of the war

Yesterday I was very angry. I can't explain why. A friend said that the 6th-7th days were the most difficult. But Yura arrived in the evening, brought some food and a disposable cig, we stayed together for a while, had a meal and tea, and I felt better. Bastia gave me a hand massage, and I gave her one too. It's relaxing. Being in the company of "my" people saves me. [...]

I am very lucky that my family has come to Lviv. Dad strongly objected to leaving early. [...] I was terribly angry with him [...] I cried for the first time because of all this, I had my first fit of hysteria. I thought that if the connection suddenly disappeared or I did not receive a response from my family and Misha, I would go crazy. This is not a figurative expression. I was sitting and shaking, feeling it with my body, I had never felt anything like that, I felt that I would go crazy in the truest sense of the word, in my mind. Rather, it seems to me that when people go crazy they feel the same way, just [multiplied by ten]. [...]

March 04

[...] I have already grazed all my nails at the roots, the skin is covered with little wounds. It's unpleasant, you have to wear plasters, and it's inconvenient to make [camouflage] nets. [...]

March 11

Today at 5:54 they hit Dnipro. Three air bombs. [...] Some places 2 km away from my house were hit. [...] I experienced all the same feelings as on the first day, I was afraid again, I had arbitrary muscle contractions again, I didn't know what to do with my hands so I just grabbed my head. Maybe this is good, because I have not felt anything for a long time. I'm not touched by the news, I'm not surprised. A kindergarten, an orphanage, a maternity hospital. All this does not cause me to be filled with proper emotions, not to mention tears. My eyes water only due to fatigue.

March 12
(From a dream diary)

[...] I dreamed that my mother and I should prepare a wedding for someone, for a woman, a friend of hers. In the dream, I did not understand who it was. And my mother had to make decorations of fresh flowers, like a garden, a landscape, roughly speaking. There were some beautiful purple flowers growing in clusters, I don't know their names. Well, in short, she had to make something of them in some locality. Then, it seems some time has passed, and we are already at this wedding. There are a lot of all kinds of people there, some are my age, some whom I don't quite know, and others, and some kind of very interesting room. And suddenly a woman runs in, she looks like some kind of Shaolin monk, she is bald, she is with a stick, and she is trying to prove something to me, to say that I cannot do something. I start arguing with her. Well, everything is clear, as if what it's all about. We start to argue, we start to fight, she is there, we run along the walls, back and forth. And in the end, she says something to me that makes me stop. She kind of knows me, she didn't seem to be going to kill me, she wanted to prove something to me. And she tells me that there is a person who wants to harm me. That person is standing nearby, a girl, too. There was also something about dolls, but I don't remember, there was some kind of point about dolls, something was wrong with those dolls, but I kind of liked them, and the woman whom I fought and me, we stop instantly, we get up from the ground, and I take her by the head, so, you know, by the face and say that you want to tell me that this is this, and this is this, and that is that, and that is that. Actually, I don't remember what I said. She says yes. And I say, damn it, exactly, thank you. And she leaves. And then, something with this girl about whom she told me everything, something is not clear, some kind of commotion begins. We start walking there, some person comes who wants to take us somewhere to swim, we all put on swimsuits and go to a river. And this river has very high banks. Rather high, well, that is, there is no beach, there is a kind of canyon and a river in it, and the canyon itself is a little bit higher than the standard pool, you know, the one you can get out of pulling yourself up with your hands. And we all swim there, and then something like fireworks starts. I think, oh, these are fireworks for the wedding, how beautiful, I look at the horizon, that is, we crawl up to the edge, climb with our hands, climb to the ground, and there is a glow over there. Lilac, lilac-pink. And I say, God, how beautiful ... are those fireworks? And the one who brought us there runs up to us and says, hide, hide, hide, do not stick out of the ditch, that one filled with water. The shelling has begun, we are hiding, and I see that I've realised that this is no longer fireworks, that this is kind of volleys being fired. [...]

And then some soldiers or policemen came and forced us to leave, lined us up and walked around for some reason, looking at us. And I really remember, I felt how tense my whole body was when I was standing at attention, because I was scared, I was trying to control myself and to stand straight. And I don't remember how it all ended. We were not shot and should be grateful even for that.

Transcribed and translated by Andrii Masliukh

Ihor K.
March 01

I was out in the city to meet a friend from Kyiv who had moved to Lviv. We talked about the feeling of guilt manifesting itself even when we do some useful, socially oriented things and help people. We talked about friends: close ones, and also about the strange pleasure of seeing photos of killed enemies. A feeling of some kind of catharsis given by the usual thought about helplessness and victim-rapist syndrome. A sense of healthy optimism. [...]

March 02

I lost 1.5 kg of weight in a few days. I currently live in a body broken by tension. [...]
   Air alarm 10:21 – 10:53am

March 03
Air alarm 1:53 – 2:36am

Another friend has gone to the military enlistment office. I worry for him. [...]
   It's calmer now. The news is calmer. I want to sleep, but this is also a reaction to a one-week-long day. [...]
   Air alarm 10:10 - 10:33am

March 04

The [situation at the] Zaporizhzhia nuclear power plant causes fear. Memories of feelings from my childhood and the panic of people in these memories. The desire to run out and to buy some iodine.
   Air alarm 9:55 – 10:11am
   [...] I've read the news about 11 women who were raped and 6 victims who died as a result. Fear again, cold in the chest. My mind paints pictures of horror.

March 05

A night without air alarms. [...]

March 06

A lot of anger and tension in the body, fatigue. [...]

March 07

It's quiet. Almost a whole day has passed without air alarms. I went downtown; where there are more people, there is more anxiety. [...]

Although I don't feel hatred now [towards the enemy], I have no kind feelings either.

March 08

The wife of a friend who serves in the police wrote to me this morning. He has not been in touch with her for a day, and she is in Poland. Later, she learned from his father that he had been sent to the frontline.

A headache, a tight chest, a sense of hopelessness, and my thoughts take on darker shades immediately. [...]

March 09

[...] [An] attack of anger, helplessness and powerlessness. [...] The desire to leave this system returns, because it cannot function like this, especially in wartime. Especially when our world is changing so quickly. Something from my past life disappears forever.

March 10

My body has given up. It couldn't stand the tension and got sick. Fatigue, stuffy nose, sore throat. Drowsiness.

A friend from Poland is going to Lviv: they want to take 12 people with them to Poland. We chatted. I smiled. I was glad to hear him.

Nazar, my friend, is already at the war. At the moment, there is no clarification as to where exactly, but he has got in touch, he is alive. [...]

March 11
Air alarm 4:43 – 4:58am

The sickness barely allowed me to wake up and go down to the shelter.

Air alarm 11:23 – 11:45am
I feel like there is a stone on my chest. I want to sleep all the time and I fall asleep instantly, finding myself in some kind of alternative history from which I cannot remember anything. [...]

There is a lot of sand-like fatigue in my body.

March 12
Air alarm 5:25 - 7:35am

It was cold. We could not wait for the alarm to be over and went to bed. [...]

March 13

[...] The seesaw of my emotional condition has now swung downwards: I don't want anything. [...]

March 14
Air alarm 2:19 – 7:41am

The father of one of my students was killed at the training ground in Novoyavorivsk.

Mykola is alive. At the time of the bombing, he was already in another place. (...)
Alarm 7:55 – 8:41am

March 15
Air alarm 11:39 – 12:44 pm

The heating was turned off for a day. Cold is very triggering. There was no air alarm at night, but I often woke up and therefore had no good night's rest. I have not much strength. Cold triggers the body to be defenceless and vulnerable, angry and aggressive. [...]

March 18
Air alarm 6:08 – 6:47am

They hit Lviv, the airport area. My folks didn't even wake up, they didn't hear anything. Dreams come back, but luckily I almost don't remember them.

Too much fatigue. Between double classes, I lie down or switch off into something like a parallel reality. It's like we have a war here, but the air still has the aftertaste of another version of history where there is no war.

March 19

I want to run away from people, especially from those close to me.

Air alarm 11:36 – 11:54am

What will happen to us if we are not active? Activism is about control. Anger is about protection, isolation is also about protection. Lack of strength to turn the world upside down and to finally heal the whole situation, with myself in it. Isolation and loneliness are what unites us. Grieving is mourning for what has been lost. We are experiencing conditions that are different, changeable and not catastrophic. If we are aware of them, they do not control us.
Air alarm 3:15 – 4:34 pm
[...]

March 22
Air alarm 6:54 – 8:20 AM

I really like to teach and learn: this is an awakening of happiness inside, which is difficult to find anywhere else now. [...]

Air alarm 1:23 – 1:35 PM; air alarm 3:17 – 4:31 PM; air alarm 5:42 – 7:50 PM; air alarm 8:31 – 9:11 PM

A desire to run away, to hide in a safe place, to isolate myself from any contact and touch. I want to wake up in a world without war, to deal with the usual, shaky reality of my trauma, not a collective one. This is too much for me alone. I don't even have the strength to cry. [...]

March 26

[...] Lviv has been bombed. I went out with my bike and immediately returned to the shelter; 10 minutes later missiles hit. I could hear it in the bathroom. The feeling of a dream that never ends intensified.
Air alarm 4:12 – 8:01 pm – 4 missiles
Air alarm 8:50 – 9:36 pm + 3 hours of meditation

March 29
Air alarm 3:46 – 4:50 am

I dreamed of my father and the Yavoriv military training ground, which my sister and I visited when we were children. Father took out his awards, showed them to me, and I asked him if his confessor had written to him, why do they cause so much suffering to the living? He replied that he [the confessor] had not written. He looked very broken and somehow desperate, in a human way. [...]

Air alarm 4:57 – 5:49 pm

Nazar is in Lviv, he came from Irpin to replace his car with a more reliable one. He gave me the records. I was very happy to hug him. He said that several hundred Grad and mortar shells fall on them every night, but he said it very calmly, as if it were his element. [...]

April 21

I want silence. I want peace and a long, long sleep. [...]
Translate by Andrii Masliukh

Sofia S.
March 03

I feel exhausted today. After 11 hours of sleep, I could barely open my eyes and force myself to wake up. It seems to be a bright return to my depressed condition, which I was lucky enough to forget for a few weeks, till this day. Well, at least it isn't the same as yesterday.

Last morning I woke up crying and started crying even harder. I had a strange dream, which I remember only in fragments. The last thing that came to my mind was writing a date on a slab and bursting into tears. The first number was "7". I hope it is March 7 — the day of the end of the war, and my tears were those of happiness. [...]

March 05

[...] It's eight p.m. and I'm at home. On the way I had to go to the grocery shop or rather to a couple of shops. I was sad and somewhat angry because I could not find most of the items on my shopping list. The shelves do not seem empty, but a lot of items are missing, and some things have almost doubled in price due to shortages. I am angry. Angry at the situation, at the world and at the injustice of life.

The house is a mess, it's cold and empty. We had to turn the heating to the maximum and to wait for 6 hours until the floor and rooms warmed up at least to a tolerable temperature. To warm myself up, I spent almost an hour sitting in a hot bath. I realized that now it is a luxury.

Life has changed and who knows if it will ever be the way it was before the war. [...]

We people are all different. There are those who flee to Poland, even from Lviv, to "save" themselves, and those who sacrifice themselves to save others. Just as there are those who are full of fear and those who are full of hatred and anger, which generates a desire to act. Among the refugees are victims who really have nowhere to go and nothing to wear, and there are those who come here in their own jeeps, rent a room in a hotel in Skhidnytsia and demand to be "served". I am sorry for the former and squeamish of the latter. [...]

Translated by Andrii Masliukh

Ruta R.
March 03

[...] I am thinking a lot about my loneliness. I feel envious seeing people supporting one another now. Maybe, I have a kind of special view of this war but I am on the frontline of my fight and I am absolutely alone. [...]

It seems to me that I will never recover after all this. Maybe, a bomb had better fall down on my head than I would feel that this war is munching me from the inside. If it lasts just a little bit longer, I will fall down like an empty shell. [...]

Since the war began, I've been having very good and quiet nightdreams. I had a nightdream of an old wonderful hotel and a temple where women were weaving colour nets; I don't remember why those were colour nets. I also had a nightdream of very green grass. Yesterday I had a nightdream that Russians were trying to invade Khortytsa. I'd spent ten years in Zaporizhzhia, and Khortytsa had been my most favourite place. If only they just have a look at Khortytsa, I will tear their eyes out. [...]

March 07

[...] My body has been becoming numb of late, the blood not reaching my extremities; they become as cold as ice all the time. It hasn't happened before. I am trying to unravel myself somehow, though I don't quite succeed: my strength evaporates with lightning speed. [...]

March 09

[...] I am feeling so upset and my soul is bleeding. I've heard someone saying that if the war ends as early as tomorrow, it will be too late. So many human lives have been lost; so many things have been ruined.

[...] I am planning to call at every church that will appear to be open, because my soul needs comforting. I am not strong enough anymore, you know. I feel a kind of helplessness. How can the world keep silent when our Ukrainian military, our Ukrainian children and our Ukrainian people are dying? How can one turn a blind eye on the fucking Russia having come to our sovereign state and having started throwing bombs on our heads and killing us? It's just outrageous. Those who are stronger would go fighting now. But I feel like crying.

[...] I wish I could fall asleep to wake up only when all this is over.

March 13

[...] Everything has evaporated: the hope, the grief and everything. What I am feeling is overall exhaustion as if I weren't alive, as if I were staying in this world just for a while. All day I've been eager to have a sleep; I don't feel like rising from bed. It's a kind of nonsense and it's unbearable. I am nervous and my body is rioting like a beast: my eyesight has become defective; I am sitting and can hardly see the letters being typed. Sometimes all my body, especially my throat and my right side feel as if pressed by something, it being uncomfortable to move. [...]

March 15

[...] So, today is Tuesday. I am feeling a kind of hope beginning to wake up. In fact, I am very thankful to all who are supporting this hope: my relatives and acquaintances, my group mates and my university instructors. I am thankful to twitter and to Arestovych after all. The phase of complete hopelessness has begun coming to an end. [...]

March 24

Today it's been a month since the war began. [...]

I've been thinking a lot that this war has taken youth from many, from millions of people. Youth is such a wonderful time but they have taken it away from us. They have taken youth away from the refugees. They have taken it away from the girls raped by the Orcs. They have taken it away from the dead. I am 17 years old now and a lot of my coevals have died. One day I will be 50 years old if I am lucky enough but they will still be 12, 15, 17. All this has happened because Russia has brought us "peace". "War is peace, freedom of slavery ignorance is power". [...]

March 25

[...] On Friday I was getting about the city and saw people, especially internally displaced people, willing to live: they were walking down the streets, eating delicious food in the restaurants, indulging in the spring wind and buying various trifles, affording to feel like tourists. I am very happy about them. We can't sacrifice our lives to death. We can't sacrifice our lives for the sake of the country; very many people are doing it nowadays. How can we forbid ourselves to live? We can't! Very often I've started seeing the thought about the military on twitter: if you can derive pleasure where there are children, do it. Don't think that you must be ashamed of doing it when a war is going on in the country and when other people are starving, suffering or dying. We can't sacrifice our lives just because some people have already sacrificed theirs: it's unwise. Those who are looking at us from the skies would be dissatisfied. It is necessary to live: so, don't be ashamed of your life. [...]

March 31

[...] I was talking about Mariupol and about the way we can witness innumerable cruel deaths that can force us to think about death. I was talking about the way we can carry on while people are dying there. And I think: we must live out of spite; we must live for the sake of life. Then I was sitting in the bathroom and crying for a long time, because I had read a story of a girl whose mother had died in Mariupol. I was reading about what she had been through, sobbing and thinking: I will live for the sake of what she has been through. I will live out of spite of death and for the sake of life. I will feel every moment of life and devote my life to those who have lost their lives; I will devote my life to those whose life broke down, whose life was broken, whose life was spoiled and ruined by the Orcs [...].

April 02-04

[...] Kyiv Region [was] freed and all that was hidden away from us is coming to us now. Before my eyes are corpses and corpses everywhere, killed or tortured Ukrainians under the banner of "Bucha Massacre". There is no getting away from these thoughts, from these images and from under-standing. [...]

April 05
(*From dream diaries*)

My mother and I went to Tartu, Estonia (Tartu is my hometown) to visit my grandfather, who owned an estate in the mountains. I must say that I don't have such a grandfather and an estate in the mountains. And there are no mountains in Tartu, but it was a nice dream. I had fun, wandered in the mountains, skated, and talked to my mom, grandpa, and dad. I walked around the city centre (for some reason, the whole city was painted over with graffiti) and ate some tasty food. It was a pleasant dream, and I was sincerely happy. I saw either a statue or a monument dedicated to hippies. [...]

I forgot to write the most important thing down. I don't remember when I had this dream, but I was in my Lviv apartment, either with my mother or with some other people. In my dream, I felt panic. There was a knock on the door. For some reason, I knew for sure the Russian soldiers were knocking. And they were knocking on with the butt of a gun. They just hit the door with their rifle butts. The dream was horrible. And not knowing what to do, we were in a fuss. We didn't even know how the armed orcs came to Lviv (to Sykhiv, to our front door!) and what they wanted. The air raid alarm woke me up. The worst nightmare I've had in wartime yet.

April 11

[...] About two hours ago, chemical weapons were thrown down on Mariupol. Probably, sarin. I am shocked; I am feeling too bad. Despair is devouring me. Who will help us anyway? Why do they let it happen? How can this cruelty fit into this world? How can we survive it? [...]

April 16

[...] The war has changed us and the space around us somewhat. It has also changed my brain: now it often passes memories and emotions through a kind of filter. All memories are falling into oblivion. They are delayed on the backroads of our memory. Our brain separates itself from traumatic experiences as hard as it can, because it has already suffered a lot. [...] Now the war has become a kind of body cross for believers: you can remember or forget that your body cross is hanging on your neck. But nevertheless, it keeps touching your naked body under your shirts, T-shirts and overcoats. The same occurs to the war: wherever I might go, no matter what kennel I might hide in, it doesn't really matter to me anymore. One can do without reminding me of my body cross, without refreshing my memory: I feel it with my naked skin all the time, all the time. This way or the other. I put up with it [...].

Translated by Mykhailo Tarapatov

Olena C.
March 06

[...] This night was a very hard one. apathy and helplessness got me; I cried and did not know what to do. it was so bad ...

March 10

[...] my mood changes all the time: from euphoria to despair [...]

today I had a dream that we defend ourselves from the Russian occupiers and won. dad said my dream was prophetic.

March 13

[...] Today, two of my favourite belarusian musicians announced a tour in russia in may. although before, I mean before the war, they claimed they wanted to play a concert in kyiv, and my friend and I were waiting for that. and now they just keep quiet about what is happening on our land and keep having fun and going to this damned russia. why now??? why when their Ukrainian fans suffer and perhaps die? why do they keep quiet? why does the whole world show solidarity and help and support, and those you considered friends or "idols" do not? it's a betrayal. I see it that way because it hurts me.

today my dad and sis had a row, and I began to notice that everyone in the family was nervous and that there was a split. it is our reaction to stress. to be honest, I can't stand it. I want to isolate myself, hide from all this despair and make everything as it was before. turn the time back. return to the time before the war. [...]

March 15

yesterday, I cried because I was afraid they could take my dad away from my sis and me. I felt so helpless and despaired; I just silently cried in the bathroom so that no one could hear me. previously I would have locked myself in my own room, but now I don't even have any personal space. I want my normal life back. I fear for my mom because there was an explosion in kyiv in the morning; I fear for my friend because military aircraft fly over her house all the time, and there are risks.

I feel exhausted

March 24

[...] today, the artillery hit a house of our co-op. the house near the house of my friend caught fire. it is 900 m from our house. I am afraid. I feel broken, so helpless. I was in a good mood this morning, and now I don't feel joy, and

I don't think I'll ever be able to again. dad says we shouldn't have bought that house. but I have so many good memories of it [...]

April 03

bucha, irpin ... these atrocities cannot be forgiven.
    "this war will go down in history as the war of those who fought for their freedom against those who fought for their slavery."
    Translated by Genyk Bieliakov

Oksana H.
Audio-visual recording
March 15, 2:05 pm

Good morning! This is the beginning of my war diaries. It is 9 a.m. sharp now. The twentieth day of the war. The night was surprisingly calm today, I woke up several times, checking my phone to see if there really were no air alarms. Now I will make tea for myself, and in two hours I'll have English. It is necessary to resume at least some studying. Our university has been destroyed. Because of that, I don't know if in the next few months or even after the war, we will return to our university. [...]. I don't know how it will all happen. But I will study English now, because I need it. I cannot say that I love this language very much, but I need it. And Ukraine will soon be in the European Union, so the need will be doubled, that's why we are to engage in self-education. No, not self-education. After all, I'm not studying this myself. And we contribute to what? Damn, it's been so long since I recorded a video.

[...] After the war started, all my emotions have been kind of blocked, I don't feel anything. There is no fear, no anger, no aggression, no panic. I have never felt so calm. I'm afraid, when it's all over, all these emotions, which are now blocked, will return to me with new strength and I will have to deal with them somehow.

Transcribed and translated by Andrii Masliukh

Kateryna L.
February 02

We sit on a time bomb. I have this feeling as if something ready to explode at any moment is actually standing close to me and breathing down my neck. [...]

February 24
Day 1

Ukraine is being bombed. Amazing. The only thing that keeps me calm is the name-mantra, which I repeat to believe in good people and their existence: "K.R., K.R., K.R ...". I saw him in a dream; I tasted the sweet and sacred feeling of warmth, harmony, and security that all his personality had instilled in me. Then I woke up, and my mother ran into my room and said that Kharkiv, Kyiv, Odessa and other cities of Ukraine were being bombed. Unlike my dream, it was very bad news. I wanted to stay in my dream so badly. Alas, the reality and all the thoughts were increasingly pushing his name out of my dreams ...

February 25
Day 2

I want to act. I want to help Ukraine. I want to give it even more strength and confidence. I'm proud. These two days have shown how strong and friendly we are; and how wonderful Ukraine and Ukrainians can be. Right now, at a time of war the likes of which, according to many, no one has seen since World War II, I say how much I LOVE THESE PEOPLE! [...]

February 27
Day 4

I can't describe this feeling when I go to bed, and my heart is pounding with anxiety when I listen to every rustle when any sound can be a siren in a nearby town or the sound of a rocket flying overhead or columns of tanks moving somewhere. I can't describe my thoughts at the moment when, already in bed, I feel the earth tremble from an unknown shock. And then, having found no signs of obvious danger around, I go back to bed, trying to calm the heartbeat and tremors in my hands, knowing that I'm falling asleep in a minefield, where anything can happen overnight. Damn Russian roulette! [...]

After a couple of days of euphoria and joy from the uprising of Ukrainians, from the fact that we made the whole world finally see us (oh, and how!), from the fact that we are ready to win, to fight for truth, dignity, and honour, after so many things we had to tell, after standing so fervently on ONE SIDE, after standing so firmly with our people, and with the whole world, there finally comes the desire to hide; you understand that you want to distance yourself from people again: it does not matter whether they are Ukrainians or foreigners; you just want to distance yourself from all the humanity, from everything that it produces, everything that it does. [...]

March 01
Day 6

[...] You don't feel strong enough to write. You don't feel strong enough to think. You can only react in a daze to the news about all the tragedies that come to life right next to you. Instead of what you loved, now there is only blood, screams, sounds of air raid alarms that blow your mind, broken windows and dilapidated houses.

Raped nation. They try to snatch the love of life from us with cruelty and tyranny. But the more pain they bring, the more the desire for life and resistance is generated.

You fall asleep, listening to every rustle, being ready for the fact that perhaps tonight hell will come to your house and you will never wake up again. Often, you hallucinate that this has already happened. You hear your relatives scream in their sleep. [...]

Each hour of this inflicts more fear. On the seventh day, this attack, which is terrible as it is, transforms more and more into a fictional story about the descent of hell to earth.

Each of these days has its specific emotional range. Today consists of an unspeakable doom. There were days when I was incredibly confident that I could hope it would end soon, when I was full of fighting spirit, when the support from the outside was so strong that it overcame all doubts. Now it is different. But it is not fear, not anxiety, it is something else ... Fatigue? Perhaps. [...]

Indifference is my biggest fear. Not pain, not anxiety, not destroyed buildings. Indifference. Because now is just the beginning, though I'm afraid it's just the tiniest bit of what can happen. But these emotions so far are fresh, ineradicable. I fear that people are getting used to the war. Going to and from the bomb shelter, news of death, bombs hitting the centres of the squares, expectations, and hope, self-defence — all this turns into a routine. When something turns into a common thing, people become indifferent. Then all emotions are blunted. People take a lot of things for granted. A lot of things lack the former expression as it was at the beginning. But this is life ... It's always like that here. [...]

March 03
Day 8

[...] Cities moan ... Their moans stab my heart. Cities howl like real living things. Cities are also hurt. They bleed in smoke. They fall apart when missiles hit them. [...]

Translated by Vitalii Pavliuk

Viktoria Y.
March 02
The seventh day

I think I'm already used to waking up to the sounds of sirens and finishing my morning coffee in the shelter. It's amazing how in 7 days, it became part of the routine of each of us. Four days ago, I shuddered at every sound or rustle, and now, every movement, every action, or thought happens automatically, without emotions. However, there is no strength or resource for emotions now.

While communicating with relatives, friends, or other people I met during volunteering, I noticed an interesting detail: our understanding of the word "good" has changed. To the question "How are you?" this answer means: "Woke up alive today. Everything is calm." [...]

March 03
The eight day

Every day the strength is decreasing. Thoughts of war and many deaths, the sound of sirens that can no longer leave my head; the feeling of powerlessness that no matter what I do, it is not enough; the feeling of shame that I am now safe, apathy and unwillingness to leave the house. It all got mixed up in an incomprehensible mix and got stuck in a lump somewhere in the throat, preventing one from thinking and acting adequately.

Today, while on duty at the volunteer headquarters, I talked with my friend about our plans after this nightmare, when we would wake up and win. A few days ago, I thought about the same thing during a sleepless night. I want to meet my friends from different regions and hug them. I want to hitchhike around all corners of Ukraine. I want to spend nights under the open sky, OUR SKY, watching the stars and how the fire burns out. I want to hang out at festivals to the music of Ukrainian artists. I want to see Crimea. I want to meet the dawn on the railway. It really has quite a therapeutic effect; these thoughts give hope that everything will be okay, that this will be over.

March 04
The ninth day

Today I woke up with the news about the attack on the Zaporizhzhia NPP. A momentary wave of anxiety. I read on - everything is fine; there is no threat of radiation spreading. I exhale with relief.

Every day it gets harder and harder to open my eyes and get out of bed. Inside, there is only a feeling of emptiness, which absorbs more and more space. Already sick of the news, sick of the constant standby mode, sick of worries. The only thing that at least somehow supports those barely burning embers is the feeling that I can help those who need it now. However, any contribution of mine seems insignificant.

March 05
The tenth day

> All that remains is a broken window, a broken cobblestone, a broken life.
> The word remains
> And in someone unchanging remains - muteness.
> The truth stands, shelled and still on guard.
> And the sun will remain, no matter what the card turns out.
> The Earth will not turn over
> It is already upside down,
> The stars are already falling from it, and with them
> and empty promises and plans collapse with a mad cry.
> Clowns rage because they are left without their masks,
> Ready to give the last
> All the same, there is nothing to lose because there are no losses.
> They walk like blind men to defeat and roll into the abyss, to their death.
> Translated by Victor Pushkar

Oksana V.
March 05

A photo from Irpyn, where civilians are hiding under the bridge from the shelling of Russian aviation. A striking photo. In this photo, we can see fear, courage, fight and invincibility at the same time. [...]

March 07

My life hasn't changed dramatically. But something new has appeared. Air raid alarms and long-lasting sirens, reading the news at night, alarm backpacks and taped windows (even though there wasn't a slightest threat of shelling), many new people and cars, taking into account that one can unmistakably tell "locals" from "commuters" in our small town by what they look like. Besides, there is MUCH more obscene language, "black jokes", hatred and horror. [...]

March 11

I've decided to start in the morning in order not to forget anything. This night was alarming from the very beginning. It is 12:39 now and the siren is still on. It is the third air raid alarm for these 24 hours; the first one was at night. We went to the corridor for the first time. It was cold and drowsy but we were not very scared. It seems to me that I will soon get used to this long-drawn roaring and that it will be my usual condition with a siren in my head. Then I couldn't fall asleep for a long time [...].

I want to write a few words about the response of my body to the war. On the first day of the war I was literally getting choked up during the first hour. When I found out about the war, I was shocked. Then it happened once again but since then, it has happened no more. During the first week of the war, a ravenous appetite woke up inside of me and I was ready to eat all I had at home. Since the war began, I've been literally immersed in sleep though a few weeks prior to that, I had problems with falling asleep. Besides, I'd always had very painful periods but the period that started on March 7th was literally THE WORST AND THE MOST PAINFUL [in] a lifetime. Medicines didn't help me. Finally, combo nimesil, two ampoules of analgen, two noshpas and a hot-water bottle produced some effect for half a day [...].

March 16

I [saw] dozens or even hundreds of photos of ruined buildings, black with soot, with smoke coming from their windows and without glazing in them. I am very sorry for those people, though [...] my sorry doesn't compare to the amount of their grief. [...]

March 18

I had a nightdream today: I saw Russian armoured vehicles in town. They were going by railway. It looked as if it were a kind of a dread locker or a tank or an armour transporting vehicle. I saw a Russian flag. A question arises: how did I see that? Did I see it while sleeping, peering from beneath a carpet or in a kind of trench or in the garden? That was a delirious nightmare but it's OK. [...]

March 20

I am already getting used to the sirens waking me up in the middle of the night. I am lucky to live in a small town which, I hope, will never be shelled or bombed, though it sometimes occurs to me that I won't live through this war the way others do [...]. It is said to be the syndrome of the one who has survived but when time comes, you become guilty because you are alive. [...]

March 22

Since today I understand that I live in a family that was suffering emotional, economic and physical violence. When people ask me how I am, they expect me to say I am all right. But I can't say that I am all right, because it's untrue. Though on the other hand, I should be glad about what I've got. If I tell them how I am, they are most likely to regret having asked, because they expected to hear "I am all right, more or less" instead and because they've apparently got nothing to help me with. [...]

March 27

It seems to me I morally or psychologically or mentally [...] burning out. I can't stand it anymore. I am permanently strained mostly because of my father who drinks like a horse. He is in a very poor condition though it is he alone who is to blame for it. I just hope we will be all right. [...]

I thought I was used to the sirens. But maybe I am not. Today I've been literally thrown up by a harsh sound. Lutsk, Zhytomyr, Kherson and other cities are being bombed. Yesterday Lviv was bombed, too. There are many people I love there. The one who is safe, the one who is sitting and waiting for at least some definite information is feeling the worst. Waiting is unbearable. [...]

April 03

[...] this day will be printed on our memories due to Bucha Massacre. This is not only Bucha. These are Hostomel, Irpyn and Mariupol ... I don't know what words I can use to express my emotions. I've already had fury, hatred, disgust and a desire for revenge. But now I am feeling helpless and I wanted to cry [...].

April 09

[...] Whatever tragedies occur, we will be mourning people, we will be sympathising with them, we will be taking revenge, growing angry and grieving. But this will not stop life; we won't stop cracking jokes, learning, listening to music and enjoying ourselves no matter what happens, because it seems like the evil done to people just stops the course of time; it seems like we will keep living the way we used to. But at the same time, I understand that nothing is capable of stopping life. And there is a kind of sorrow and happiness at the same time. And there is more happiness than sorrow here. [...]

April 12

[...] In one of the diaries I read a quotation from Bohdan S.: we must get up, live, breathe, talk, hug and kiss one another. I understand it like living at full force without waiting for better times and enduring hard times, because no one knows what will be tomorrow; there is only today and we must live it as best as we can.

April 17

[Katia and I went for a walk and we] were talking about what was important now. We were talking about how we'd met the war, about how it had changed us and about the relations we've got now. Each of us bought herself a bunch of narcissuses. We called at a nice coffee house, a very atmospheric one. She took some pictures of me [and] told me that I was beautiful [...]. We must give ourselves these small presents, the reasons to be happy: the flowers presented to ourselves, visits to a coffee house and walks even if it is not sunny and even if it is very windy. Even at the time of the war. I haven't been so glad for a long time. I feel I am living and that's wonderful. [...]
    Translated by Mykhailo Tarapatov

Polina S.
February 24
6:37 am

Probably the scariest thing you can hear in your life is the words, "Wake up, we're under attack."

These words marked my February 24, 6:37 a.m. A worried mother, in a hurry, not believing in her own words, repeats this line to me thrice. I jump up from my two-story bed, look at my younger brother, who is still sleeping so sweetly, and ask again, as if it were a dream, as if it couldn't be real, "What? Who? How?". Although, the answer to these questions was obvious.

They started bombing Ukraine, including my hometown Kyiv, at 5 in the morning, insidiously, while everyone was sleeping. But my mother did not wake me up; she never tried to wake me up early, even in a critical situation. I immediately pick up the phone (what a bad habit to do this in the very morning) and see a bunch of messages from my friend, "POLINA, WE WERE ATTACKED, WE WOKE UP FROM THE EXPLOSIONS." I open the news feed, and then the world ceased to exist. I do not believe; I do not accept the *new* truth, and I do not want to believe in it.

However, my body is already shaking so much that I just can't keep myself on my feet. And I wouldn't say that I was shaking with fear, no. If I was worried, I was most afraid not even for my life but for the future of my country. Will we be captured? Will the suffering of our ancestors and all that they fought for be in vain? Everything looked consistent in my head: there will be no country, no future for my people and my family. [...]

I heard explosions that day. The first explosions in my life, in my hometown. I remember my impressions and the lack of perception of the situation that happened in Donetsk, Luhansk in 2014: you know that this is happening to your Ukraine, to people, to your friends there, but you do not perceive it as something real. Yes, it is there, but somewhere far away, it will definitely not come to you. And when it comes to you, only then do you realise all the horror, the horror of war.

But the worst was at night: you have trouble falling asleep because of the incessant flow of thoughts, your whole body trembles, and you never know *where* the next rocket will hit. Maybe our house?

I tried to go to bed earlier, to fall asleep, desperately, to rest, but it never happened. And when it did, you would wake up in the middle of the night to the explosions, which now sounded even closer to our house. It was the first day. The first day when everything turned upside down.

March 13-14
(From a dream diary)

After we left Kyiv, and then the Kyiv region, where we had lived for more than a week since the beginning of the war, constantly hearing sounds of explosions and fighter jets, and when we found relative safety in Uzhhorod, I had my first dream with a "plot". [...]

The dream felt very real. There I was again in the village, near our house, where we had spent the first week of the war — the village of Ustymivka, near Bila Tserkva.

However, it was exactly an apocalyptic dimension, as if something very bad had happened to Ukraine, and I did not know what exactly. I felt anxiety and real fear every second. Ash flew in the air, everything around was very grey and empty, and dusk was about to settle in that small village.

I remember hiding all day behind a "concrete blockade" with some guys and girls I had never met before, but I knew for sure that they were my people and we should be together. I had my dog, the Yorkshire Terrier Mira, with me.

However, in the evening, apart from dusk, something very, very scary was coming, and at one moment, we somehow understood it all together. Honestly, I don't remember what happened, but all the guys shouted: "To the shelter! Everyone, go home!" There was no need to repeat it twice. Mira and I ran to our house. I noticed the improvised "blockade" was right in front of my house ... Why?

The house, which our family always called "hut" because it was quite old and abandoned even before the war, and we came there infrequently, was almost totally bombed. There was no water, no light, no gas, but for some reason, the windows survived.

I took the dog in my arms and came carefully in. I remember looking anxiously out of the windows, and all the time, I felt someone incredibly dangerous was walking on the street. It was a feeling when you're afraid to breathe so that no one can hear or see you, knowing otherwise they'll just kill you. I thought of the people I saw at the checkpoint: were they alive? were they safe?

At that moment, my dream ended. [...] I analysed and asked: "Where are my parents? Where are my uncle and grandma, who used to live in this house?" However, I just couldn't find the answers — I went further in my dream to survive.

Translated by Yulia Kulish

Iryna B.
(From a dream diary)

Tight hugs. [...] It's the first thing I remember from my dream. Then there were more hugs, packing my backpack and bags in a small light room. Somehow, everyone I said goodbye to left earlier, and I kept trying to check if I had packed everything I needed and put it on my shoulders conveniently. I spent much time packing, a bit too much, until I started to panic that nobody would be waiting for me outside.

Indeed, no one was outside, but I took it for granted. Space around me reminded me of the exit from the *Dnipro* metro station in Kyiv. And when I went in the direction of the river, my sister was next to me. The surroundings changed again. There was no river anymore, just a bit of it beyond the tree rows. We argued which road to follow. The one along the riverbank was full of the spring rains, and people had to balance on the thin, dry ground line between the road, trees, and riverbank. No cars were there, but if they were, they would splash water over pedestrians. The other road passed through the tree rows, away from the puddles and the Dnipro. It was a sunny Spring day. [...] [The] dream was interrupted. [...]

Translated by Viltalii Pavliuk

Kateryna R.
February 25

The war has begun. It's been on for two days already. Everyone is running somewhere or doing something: collecting humanitarian aid, weaving masking nets or writing letters to the military. I don't want to do anything; I just want to sleep. I am ashamed of having no desire to help. [...] I want to close myself down. In spite of this, I go with my friends to weave masking nets and to write letters. I'VE GOT to do something. Everybody is doing something. [...]

March 03

Poland. Today I've noticed how much the war has changed me. [...]

March 04

Shame. At night a friend of mine who is in Cherkasy, Ukraine now telephoned me. [...] [She] was crying and said that her parents had decided to send her, her mother and her sister to Poland. She said that she was ashamed of having to go and that she didn't want to. [...] [She] wanted to help here, in Ukraine, instead of running away.

March 05
Sirens.

I am staying with my father's friends in Poland. Their home is situated near a fire brigade station. When somebody's house is on fire, the fire brigade station summons all its workers with a loud SIREN heard all over the town. I was warned that it was not an air raid alarm. But my heart sinks when I hear that sound. [...] Every time the sirens roared, I thought that the town was about to be bombed. Now I can't calm down. [...]

March 09

Today Instagram was full of photos of the maternity hospital in Mariupol. Russians had hit it, there being 17 sufferers. I am looking at the photos, where there are pregnant mothers with blood on their heads, where a very pale woman is being carried; she is either pregnant or already dead. I become numb with this news. [...]

March 21

Hrytsak said: "We shouldn't build illusions for ourselves: this war won't be quick to end". I want to go home. I don't want this war to last months or years. I want to be with my family on Easter. Do I really have to live in

Poland, earning money, looking for a place to live in and to get on with life? I don't want it; I am staying here just for a while.

Let the war end, please!

March 24

I talked with my father via video connection. I had never been so close to him before. I am used to not showing emotions. Dad was lying in a barrack, where there were many beds, with a military uniform on. The beds were arranged one above another. He asked how I was doing and if I had made friends in Poland. Dad said that after the war we would tour Poland all together and do the sights.

We finished the video connection. Now I am sitting and crying. It hurts me too much to see my father with a military uniform on [...]. Life is splitting into pieces. [...]

March 29

I had a nightdream of Cherkasy, my home city. When I was asleep, I was walking down familiar streets and feeling at home. I was watching spring coming to my city. I was so glad! Because of that nightdream, I didn't feel like waking up; I wanted to stay a little bit longer [...].

Translated by Mykhailo Tarapatov

Yevheniia M.

It seems I have forgotten what life is and how to live. Emotions turned off the first day; I don't cry. I'm cold and emotionless. It's probably worse than sobbing for days. I don't seem to feel anything anymore, only anger. [...]

War is primarily a shock. It's a shock connected with the thing that once someone destroyed the entire reality that you so accurately built brick by brick. Everything was not perfect; there was still a lot of work, but now an escalator demolished everything; now there is level ground again. It's hard to accept, it's hard to find yourself in all this and do at least something. The first association with the land now is the pictures of the bodies of Russian soldiers, whom the land embraces.

My Sonya is somewhere in the basements of Severodonetsk, among mines, saboteurs, and food that is running out. [...]

Music helps. Mostly after listening, I want to find a gun and shoot, but I know that these are extremes, I can't do it. And I was always a pacifist.

The whole day consists of reading the news and talking with friends. How is it in Kharkiv, Kyiv, Volnovakha, Mariupol and Lviv? Is everyone alive and well? Fine. Now all that remains is to blame me for not being under fire. [...]

Translated by Yulia Kulish

Oksana D.
February 24

I got up from the sound of sirens (martial law). Then I opened the news and could not stop. The war began. Anxiety gripped my body; I felt my heart jump out of my chest. I wrote to relatives who were in Chernivtsi. They are fine. Missiles hit almost every city.

It was Thursday, the day of challenging seminars I had been preparing for the previous days. Now Thursday is associated with the beginning, with the first day. It was the hardest emotionally. I tried to do everything as usual. Although, at first, I collected an alarm backpack [*tryvozhna sumka*] with the necessary. I went to the store (there was terrible excitement) and went to the New Post Office [*Nova Poshta*] because my parents had sent me food the day before. Then I walked around campus. We ordered a pizza with a roommate (that day, La Piez collected all the money for the order at the Armed Forces) and watched the cartoon "Soul". I constantly read the news. I passed the deadline in my English classes. Recorded the video in Spanish. In short, I tried to live my life. [...]

March 03

Yesterday in Chernivtsi, there was a siren three times: in the morning, in the evening, and at 2 at night. That night was terrifying. I was shaking, and I had pain in my chest. And when there was an evening alarm, the rocket hit the south station in Kyiv ... BASTARDS DEGENERATES THE STATION FUCK, WHERE A LOT OF PEOPLE, THEY BLASTED INTO THE HEATING SYSTEM, WHICH COULD MAKE PEOPLE STAY IN COLD HOMES
I HATE, I WANT TO SHOUT
I'm tired of the news; I'm tired of the war
I'm safe (physically), but it's hard for me too [...]

March 09

14 days since the beginning of this hell
the news about the mass grave in Mariupol killed me
the information that virtually all of Mariupol was held hostage shocked me when I realized it
more than a thousand civilians have died in Mariupol since the beginning of this hell
Fuck
I was in Mariupol three years ago
it was a European city that was developing, where investments poured in, and where the president came to meet with entrepreneurs
it hurts [...]

March 21

in a dream, a tank's barrel (?) was directed at my car. I managed to save myself and then ran away from the Muscovite, and we got into a fight; and I skewered him and then waited for him to die ... a good friend of mine turned out to be a Muscovite, but I still wanted him to die [...]

May 07

Yesterday I drove my family home by car about 10 minutes before curfew. The city was already dark. Street lights are off.

To protect yourself, you must become invisible. Every night in Ukraine, cities hide in the dark to become invisible.

Like a game with a small child:

Where is Ukraine?
turns off the light
There is no Ukraine
turns on the light
Here is Ukraine!
turns off the light
And where is Ukraine? No Ukraine?
turns on the light
Aha, this is where Ukraine is!
turns off the light
And where is Ukraine? No Ukraine?
turns on the light [...]
Translated by Viktor Pushkar

Mariia K.
February 24
Lera, Stefa, Sasha

I:	Lera, what day is today?
Lera:	The first day of the war.
I:	How happy we are!
Stefa:	Almost like the first day of spring!
Lera:	We are sitting, everything is fine, we're hugging each other and hardly crying. They say we can be bombed today.
I:	Oh! What time is it now?
Stefa:	23:28. We keep reading the news every 15 seconds.
Lera:	That's great.
I:	I have a few questions, the first is how was your morning today?
Stefa:	Unforgettable.
Sasha:	You know, [we felt] very much together, all three of us were thinking before going to bed, God, what is it like to get up in the morning for those two workshops? But, you know, waking up with a siren is very, very convenient. Because you wake up feeling like you never want to sleep in your life.
Lera:	In general, it is an interesting experience, of course, but I don't think anyone should live it.
Stefa:	In Russia.
Lera:	Let them worry in Russia. Amen. [...]
Stefa:	Let them experience all the anxiety that I experienced for a whole day, in every second.
I:	Do you have any feelings about this event?
Lera:	This event ... I don't know, I'm afraid for everyone very much. And even a little today, but there is some hope that ours ... Sorry, just news here: "Russia has deployed more than 60 battalion tactical groups in Ukraine", a message from the headquarters. [...]
I:	Sasha, how are you feeling today?
Sasha:	I realized two things in regard to our condition, firstly, you prioritize very well, because when I was packing my bag, I was like, well, okay, I see now how much stuff I don't need, secondly, you realize how many people you really love. Even those whom you seemingly hate. [...]
I:	And one last question, we are now finishing our mini interview. Your predictions: how long will all this take place?
Stefa:	Until the Russians die out.
I:	So long?
Lera:	I don't know, I don't think it's a blitzkrieg, because it's already obvious that it's not a blitzkrieg. Because they would have seized

everything in one day, a lot of. But, honestly, I don't think that it will be very long.

I: And how long?

Lera: I just understand that it depends a lot on how they will destabilize the situation, if they bomb, it might be soon enough. Or if they drive the government out, then I think it will be soon enough. But again, it's like no one can ...

I: According to your feelings, will it be long, not long?

Valeria: Honestly, it seems like long, but I hope they ...

I: Longer than a month?

Valeria: Yes. [...]

Transcribed and Translated by Andrii Masliukh

PART II

The Ruptures and Ruins of War

4

DREAMING OF WAR

Stephen Frosh

Dreamscapes

When war comes, the world closes in. Sirens wail. In the diaries and dreams created and reported by students and academics in the first two months of the Russian invasion of Ukraine in 2022, which construct a kind of dreamscape of the war, it seems like it is the sirens that speak loudest to the (mostly) young women who record their responses; women who are anxious about their families and their lovers, who are displaced or sheltering, who have found it hard to believe that such things as these can happen in reality, to their homes and in their country. The sirens break into psychic life everywhere. Sirens wake Sofia D. from her dream of February 11 in which she is standing amidst a mass of little mice that she feels are crawling over her.

> At night I also dreamed, I don't remember exactly, but I remember that there were a lot of … in short, I was standing somewhere and there was one mouse and a lot of little mice. But the little mice are so small, like, you know, newly-born kangaroos, they were just running around like fleas … like some bugs, in general. There were so many of them, and they were running around. And at first, I was afraid that I would step on them because I really stepped on one, you know, it was someone's mouse, not just a conditional rat. It was someone's mouse, someone else was standing next to me trying to calm me down. And then there were so many of them that I started to panic, I started to run away from them. I felt like they were crawling over me, so I started to shake them off, to walk around, and all that. And then I was woken up by the siren.

DOI: 10.4324/9781003449096-8

For Oksana D. sirens 'howl' and it is ants rather than mice that come to mind: 'It's scary to run out into the basement at night. Then nothing can be seen, only the howling of sirens can be heard. I then imagine the invisible city coming to life. As if thousands of tiny ants run out of their homes and go to the storage rooms' (May 07). Mariana H. is 'afraid to go to the shower, wash my head, cook buckwheat, go outside—sirens wail everywhere, alarm, you have to run, escape. Panic inside, a "poker face" outside. And everyone is tired of the words: "Everything is fine, I understand you"' (February 26, p. 207). The sirens belie the attempt at reassurance. Everything is *not* fine and other people's hasty 'understanding' of what each individual is going through is inadequate or misplaced. Mariana H. writes, 'It seems I lived the previous days on adrenaline only. Today, I began to fully understand what is happening. In place of adrenaline a total exhaustion came. I can't put myself in order; the usual routine has been replaced by the ritual of scrolling news' (February 27, p. 207).

Everyone is in much the same situation, yet each person's experience is different; holding on to this singularity is an important marker of sustained subjective being. Anastasiia B. also cannot stay in the shower for more than a couple of minutes in case the sirens interrupt her, and eventually the frequency of the sirens wears her out. 'And at some point,' she writes 'I just didn't care anymore. I pretended there was no siren, and I tried to keep doing what I was doing while thinking, "nothing will hit our house, that's for sure"' (March 22). Her self-reassurance perhaps keeps her going, but it is a flimsy protection both against the real bombs outside and in terms of preserving a calm state of mind. On the night of the 9th to 10th March, for example, after a couple of days that have been siren-free, she is sheltering and feeling more secure; the return of the sirens is devastating.

> I'm sitting in a bathroom with my parents and little sister. Air-raid sirens have been wailing for 10 minutes straight. It's scary to listen to their nervous and intermittent breathing. At the collegium in the bunker, everyone's trying to distract themselves somehow. Here, there is silence, breathing, darkness, and this air-raid siren. The town is small, and one can hear all of them. The siren echo builds itself up. It's been a couple of days without the sirens. One gets used to good things quickly. I was overwhelmed by the last siren, as if it was the first one. (Anastasiia B., March 10, p. 199–200)

'It's scary to listen to their nervous and intermittent breathing': does this refer to her parents and her sister or to the sirens themselves? Do sirens breathe? Breathlessness is another feature, the sucking out of air, gasping for a freer life. 'I can't breathe,' reports Yelyzaveta B. of a premonitory dream from just before the war, 'it's dark before my eyes, and I don't understand why it's so dark for so long. Perhaps the whole after-death thing will be like this: darkness and uncomfortable pressure in the chest' (recorded on March 28, p. 216). Anastasiia I. too, in a dream of vulnerability and near-death, focuses on breath, either as a moment of hope or of resignation: 'I take one last deep breath and exhale as slowly as I can. It seems I can live on this exhale for at least another day of my life. Even for an eternity' (April 25, p. 234). 'I can't breathe' has become a contemporary motif for oppression, a rallying cry at times, but also a marker of violent death. Here it arises naturally and symptomatically in dreams. Yet it also expresses something to hold in mind with these dreams and diaries: the *whiteness* of the reports. 'I can't breathe' comes from the Black Lives Matter movement, its relaying of the experience of Black lives especially in America, but elsewhere too. In the reception of Ukrainian refugees, there has been discrimination between Black and White; and in the UK and other countries, the contrast between the attitude taken towards Ukrainians in comparison with that towards black and brown refugees and migrants has been stark, especially at the governmental level. The breathlessness reported in these dreams and diaries does not consciously reference this racism, yet it evokes it, a reminder of the selectivity in suffering, the way the structures of racism insinuate themselves everywhere.

Anastasiia I. holds onto a piece of reality in relation to the sirens, but also notices the processes of denial:

While the sirens wail, I sit in the bathroom. In a cold bathroom with the lights off because only there do I have a bit of personal space and hope that I won't be in so much pain if they hit my house. In Drohobych, everyone ignores sirens, and I no longer have the strength to persuade them to at least turn the lights off in the evening. I just go to the bathroom and cry while they believe in eternal luck. Yes, everyone is already thinking I'm a crazy one who always worries in vain. But I know it's just until the first casualty in the town. (March 14)

Oksana V. hears the sirens as a 'roar'. She states on March 11, 'It seems to me that I will soon get used to this long-drawn roaring and that it will be my usual condition with a siren in my head' (p. 85). Yet presumably precisely because it has become her 'usual condition', it does not go away, but neither does she really get used to it; the sirens 'roar' throughout her diary. Anastasiia B. helps us to understand some of this through the summary account of 'Senses through War' that opens her diary, under the heading, 'Hearing':

- What is the way to not hear an air-raid siren or a missile whistling in every sound?
- Why is it so essential to control the noise space? In which way does every additional sound affect the collective nervous system?
- Sound affects body movement; we freeze like panthers at every rustle. But our poacher is treacherous; he can shell you from above.

Not hearing; controlling the noise space to protect the 'collective nervous system'; freezing but then being exposed to the shells from above. The evocation here is of a traumatic encounter; the sirens are not simply signals of encroaching danger—a realistic focus for fear or 'signal anxiety' (Skelton, 2006)—nor do they *represent* anything in the dreams and diaries. Instead, they constitute a direct incursion on the psyche; they *are* the trauma. Defending against these sirens through denial ('I pretended there was no siren', as Anastasiia B. writes in the extract given above) is a conscious, self-aware process that no-one really believes will work; in the end, the siren is 'overwhelming'. Yet there is a self-protective impulse at work here, mobilised by anger and anxiety, a refusal to give in to the intrusion and become traumatised. It is important not to hear 'a missile whistling in every sound' (Anastasiia B).

These sirens warn of attack and so are aimed at protecting the population, yet they themselves have a traumatising impact, carrying the weight of the aggression and penetrating the psychic life of the dreamer/diarist. They infiltrate or disturb dreams, they spread so that there can be no escape from the war. They make it immanent; sound penetrates in ways that are much harder to resist than that of the other senses. Closing one's ears is more difficult than closing one's eyes. The auditory register of war is what gets inside the writers, making them experience it even when physically they are apparently unscathed. Even in the shelters, the sirens can be heard; and the darkness there makes it harder to know what the reality of bombing outside might be. Sirens create the anxiety that is attached to what they warn against, so that what should be (and in reality is) a protective warning becomes itself an assailant. This is akin to the splits and dissensions that happen within families, also documented in some of the diaries: those who one cares about most, and are most anxious for, can become a source of tension. Yelyzaveta B. writes in her diary of March 02:

Today I am 20. I've been living in Lviv for 4 years but I am not afraid to offend my family with my point of view, because the internal truth can't be hushed up or ignored. N says that I've already grown up for the time of learning and that I understand the things they will never be able to understand. I am crying in the bathroom with his words, because these thoughts appear and these fears are becoming real and filling the space all around: inside my family, misunderstanding outgrew the tastes in music or in movies. And it was becoming scarier, deeper and harder. The people who have grown me up don't understand me. But I understand myself. I in no way doubt myself and my view, the view that I am not alone. I am never alone.

Yelyzaveta B. has stronger and clearer views on the invasion than her parents; they neither understand her nor fully respect her ideas, so she feels alienated from them. Others too recount their irritation with their families amongst their fears, their sense of loss and distance mixed sometimes with anger and often with an observable loneliness. Olena C. writes on March 13:

[T]oday my dad and sis had a row, and I began to notice that everyone in the family was nervous and that there was a split. It is our reaction to stress. To be honest, I can't stand it. I want to isolate myself, hide from all this despair and make everything as it was before. (p. 77)

For Oksana V., the war brings into focus the pre-existing troubles in her family, including her father's alcoholism, and the fact that no one can help:

Since today I understand that I live in a family that was suffering emotional, economic and physical violence. When people ask me how I am, they expect me to say I am all right. But I can't say that I am all right, because it's untrue. Though on the other hand, I should be glad about what I've got. If I tell them how I am, they are most likely to regret having asked, because they expected to hear "I am all right, more or less" instead and because they've apparently got nothing to help me with. (March 22, p. 86)

Oksana V. understands that she is not all right but the war insists on everyone claiming to be all right, because no one has the resources to help those who are not. 'Everything is fine, I understand you' is a lie.

Of course, most of the anger is against Russia, a visceral anger that spares no one and is linked to a sense of betrayal as well as a rise in patriotism. How can the Belorussian bands that Olena C. favours dare to perform in Russia (March 13, p. 77)?

They just keep quiet about what is happening on our land and keep having fun and going to this damned Russia. Why now??? why when their Ukrainian fans suffer and perhaps die? why do they keep quiet? why does the whole world show solidarity and help and support, and those you considered friends or "idols" do not? It's a betrayal. I see it that way because it hurts me.

Betrayal and lack of trust: in Anastasiia B.'s dreams of 12th March, eventually disrupted by the siren, she is in the doctor's waiting room but is aware that the doctor 'slyly' intends to do her harm; and then, her father is hurting her sister. 'The doctor and dad are the people I trust,' she writes, 'they help me, they wish me best. But in these dreams, they hurt me, and I'm afraid of them' (March 12, p. 200–201). The paranoid state of mind here is a reflection of the persecutory world, but it infects everything, even those who are the people one (usually) trusts. Mariana H. finds herself unexpectedly dreaming on March 10, this time a brutal dream:

For the first time in six months, I had a dream. I sat in Zelensky's office while he read something carefully. I thought he needed support like no one else. I couldn't think of anything better and decided to just give him a hug. He said I should leave because they were going to record his video address. I politely left. At that moment, I saw a crowd of extras coming into the office. "Why can't I be there?" I stood aside. Zelensky confidently said something to the camera, and suddenly Russian military men with machine guns burst into the room. They shoot everywhere, at everyone, those bastards. While I fall to the ground to hide, the extras are petrified, and the president continues to read his address. Through my fingers, I notice that the faces of those murderers are not just faces but holograms. It seems that Putin's face is superimposed on the face of each soldier; they either mix or overlap each other; it's scary. Like a large army of one man. Recently I learned that Putin has doppelgangers. Maybe that's who they are? I'm trying to fight off the bullets; I don't know what to do … "Good morning! Get up!! Polya leaves for Georgia". (p. 208–209)

Much of this material seems transparent, reflecting the realistic anxiety and suffering of the dreamers and diary-keepers, their anger and emotional turmoil, their exhaustion and fear for the present and the future, their incomprehension and sense of betrayal. Occasionally, they draw on past history to solidify their hatred of Russia and Russians (who are in places referred to as 'orcs'): for example, both Zhenia T. and Oksana V. reference the Holdomor, the Great Famine perpetrated by Stalin's Soviet Union on Ukraine, which killed millions of people in the 1930s (p. 54). There are escape dreams, dreams of rescue and triumph, expectations of victory and overt wish fulfilments. There is also realistic, even ironic, reflection on the impact of the war on everyday life and the simple exchanges of relationality. Viktoria Y. writes on March 02:

While communicating with relatives, friends, or other people I met during volunteering, I noticed an interesting detail: our understanding of the word "good" has changed. To the question "How are you?" this answer means: "Woke up alive today. Everything is calm." And only after hearing this "good", which means very little in peacetime, one breathes a sigh of relief. (p. 83)

On March 22, Anastasiia I. writes about mourning her future in a way that almost certainly embraces other young people's experiences as well:

> And then I realized I have been in a deep mourning for some time now. I have been in a real mourning for the future, which will definitely never be the way I imagined it (because now I'm really afraid to plan anything), and for the past too, which will never be the way it seemed to go on forever. After all, they just shot my past and future down. And now I have to live with this emptiness in my chest. I have to live with this hole, through which the wind sings and even rain drops; sometimes crumbs of food and other trash fall there, but nothing can fill it anymore because the loss is too vast. It has hit me through. (p. 234)

Both future and past have to be mourned; the destruction of hope and memory leaves an aching void. And Zhenia T.'s words, in one of her last diary entries on April 05, links precisely with this sense of mourning and loss:

> I remember the time when I wasn't afraid to remain silent and think for a couple of hours very well. The time when one doesn't have to flee to the imaginary better worlds. I used to have my own one. Now, my world is inferior, shaky, dark, and bizarre—it's like an empty city after the bombing. (p. 56)

An empty city after the bombing: this seems very close to one of the most powerful Freudian notions, developed in the midst of a war a century ago: melancholia.

The War Inside

The Russian invasion of Ukraine is not the first war to have taken place since psychoanalysis was invented. The catastrophic European wars of the twentieth century were in many ways a breeding ground for psychoanalytic ideas and practices and for magnifying psychoanalysis' impact (Shapira, 2013). In particular, it is arguable that these wars served to redirect the focus of psychoanalysis away from the management of desire and sexual impulses (the main topic of early Freudian work, especially in relation to hysteria and phobias) and towards questions of intimacy and, especially, loss. Such a claim cannot be universally upheld, with Lacanian psychoanalysis in particular mounting an assault on the retreat from Freudian purity entailed by the move towards intersubjectivity and relationality that characterises so much of the contemporary psychoanalytic world. Nevertheless, it does seem to be a reasonable characterisation of shifts in psychoanalysis over the period: from drive to object relations, from one-person to two-person systems, from subject-object to what Jessica Benjamin (1998) calls 'subject-subject psychology'; and from ontology to relationality (Butler, 2012). This can be persuasively traced to the shift in Freud's own thinking during and after the First World War, although this was complex and in some ways ambiguous and self-contradictory; it can be seen more clearly in the arrival of Kleinian and object relations thinking in Britain, the emergence of relational and intersubjective thought in the USA, and the spread of a general concern about loss and mourning throughout the psychoanalytic world, linked especially to the impact of war. The rise of the Kleinian 'depressive position' is an indicator of this, but so is the more recent interest in melancholia, including in relation to gender and postcolonialism. It can also be seen, as Michal Shapira (2013) shows, in the increased psycho-analytic and social policy concern with child development and the necessary conditions for attachment, security and intimacy that ought to be provided by a stable, caring society – and that are frequently disrupted by ongoing privation and violence.

This is not the place for a review of this voluminous material (see Frosh, 1999), though it is worth noting that the capacity of psychoanalysis to respond to the reality of war by developing new concepts attuned to experiences of loss and destruction is some evidence of its sensitivity to 'external', social issues and a riposte to the widespread criticism that it reduces human experience to psychological states, that it is too rigid and inwardly focused. Psychoanalysis has stayed alive and relevant because it has been able to respond to new features of the world, to the actual problematics of people's existence and the troubles they bring with them to the consulting room and to the social ramifications of these experiences. The external environment demands such responses and psychoanalysis has always had a capacity to offer some, however haltingly at times. For Freud, an early reaction to the First World War was to make important distinctions between different kinds of anxious fearfulness, especially between those that have a realistic object and those that are generalised too far. In *Beyond the Pleasure Principle*, he distinguishes between different types of emotional responses to danger. Discussing the various terms one might use to name these, he comments,

> 'Fright', 'fear' and 'anxiety' [in German, 'Schreck', 'Furcht' and 'Angst'] are improperly used as synonymous expressions; they are in fact capable of clear distinction in their relation to danger. 'Anxiety' describes a

particular state of expecting the danger or preparing for it, even though it may be an unknown one. 'Fear' requires a definite object of which to be afraid. 'Fright', however, is the name we give to the state a person gets into when he has run into danger without being prepared for it; it emphasizes the factor of surprise. (Freud, 1920/1955, p. 12)

Freud makes it clear that anxiety is an *adaptive* response to danger, mobilising the defences against it. Anxiety can get out of hand, but in principle it is necessary; without it, one would fall prey to the danger itself, with no preparation. Fear, too, is generally speaking adaptive: it knows what the danger is and reacts to it. But *fright* (Schreck) is a different state altogether. Fright is what we get when we are unprepared for the danger we have encountered. Sometimes this is necessary, in an odd way, to stave off anxiety. For example, Freud (1920/1955) suggests that certain unpleasant dreams might serve the function of raising anxiety in the dreamer precisely in order to make it possible for a danger to be recognised. If we are afflicted by a trauma, a problem we have is to symbolise in the face of the difficulty of articulating what it is we are troubled by. The dream points to the thing that cannot be said and finds a way to represent it. It repeats this representation until it is heard, until anxiety is generated—because once we feel anxious, it may become possible to defend ourselves against the frightening thing. So sometimes we seek out danger in order to clarify what we are afraid of, because once that happens—once the feared object can be symbolised—we might be able to survive it.

In the case of the Ukrainian dreams and diaries, there is not much evidence of actively seeking out danger but running 'into danger without being prepared for it' is certainly part of the story. Even with all the sabre-rattling that preceded the Russian invasion, there was plenty of denial, or perhaps just the hope that nothing would come of it. Part of the shock of Schreck is precisely this willed unexpectedness. But there is more evidence of 'Furcht' and 'Angst', fear with a specific object in mind, and anxiety with a generalised one. The anxiously melancholic reverberations of the dream and diary sequences described previously resonate strongly here: persecutory intrusion by sirens warning of bombing; anger and hatred toward the aggressor; splits and fractiousness in intimate relationships; anxiety bearing down on one so that people find it hard to breathe; loss of loved ones, loss of one's past through the destruction of homes and cities and the revelation of the illusory nature of any sense of security; loss of the future through these young people's realisation that they will be displaced, that their plans and visions for themselves will have to be fundamentally rethought. There is much that psychoanalysis might say about this that does not involve reducing these experiences to neurotic anxieties, but rather recognises their sources in the actual materiality of the warring world. This world both expresses and gives rise to certain psychic states. The violence of war becomes the backdrop to subjective reality, so that the fantasies that inform dreams and the relatively unconstrained ruminations that are mobilised in diary writing, are themselves indicators of that violence. As Jacqueline Rose (1996, p. 5) testified some time ago in her discussion of how 'like blood, fantasy is thicker than water,' subjective and material reality are indissociable, meaning not that they determine one another, but that they dance in tune.

For Freud, the First World War was a time for reflections on melancholia, trauma and death. His most important statement on the former, *Mourning and Melancholia* (Freud, 1917/1957) understood it as a process linked with failed mourning. He wrote, now famously,

> The distinguishing mental features of melancholia are a profoundly painful dejection, cessation of interest in the outside world, loss of the capacity to love, inhibition of all activity, and a lowering of the self-regarding feelings to a degree that finds utterance in self-reproaches and self-revilings, and culminates in a delusional expectation of punishment. This picture becomes a little more intelligible when we consider that, with one exception, the same traits are met with in mourning. The disturbance of self-regard is absent in mourning; but otherwise the features are the same. (Freud, 1917/1957, p. 244)

Freud understands that successful mourning requires acceptance of loss and a gradual losing of that loss, so it becomes a thing of the past; melancholia is a kind of failed mourning, made difficult because of the resistance on the part of the subject to acknowledging that loss has occurred at all—the lost object was, in fantasy, '"never" loved and "never" grieved', as Butler (1997, p.34) puts it in her retelling of the story in the context of gender melancholy. But in the Ukrainian situation, how can something be despatched to the past when it is continuing with such literal force in the present? There is nothing 'post-traumatic' about this, as the traumatic experience drags on; the loss and fear of loss cannot be resolved as a memory if it remains present, if the losing is continuous. Zhenia T.'s description of her 'world' as 'inferior, shaky, dark, and bizarre—it's like an empty city after the bombing' (April 05, p. 56) comes to mind. Something has been emptied out, or bombed to nothingness, leaving ruins and a melancholic substructure. It can be mourned, but not yet, because its emptiness has not been fully processed, because the 'lostness' of the treasured thing is not yet past. The loss is in the present as the bombing continues, each new siren bringing it back into consciousness, into a kind of life in which the losses mount up. The problem of the empty city after bombing is that reconstruction cannot occur whilst the bombs continue to fall. 'How do we memorialize an event that is still ongoing?' asks Christina Sharpe (2016, p. 20) in her very different context, but still one of violence. For her, slavery translates into the ongoing disaster of antiblack racism, which as noted earlier has been visible in the response to the Ukrainian crisis. But generally, there is no final 'coming to terms with' continuing atrocity—an issue that has been of practical concern in many contexts and amongst other things has given rise to truth and reconciliation commissions in various places and to a large psychoanalytically informed literature on recognition and forgiveness. How can memorialising or even mourning occur to fix a loss in place when the loss goes on, renewed all the time?

Melancholia is preserved because mourning cannot take place under conditions of continued bombardment. Loss of hope is as poignant as loss of place, perhaps not as searing as loss of loved persons, but still powerful enough and connected to the realistic sense that no one and nothing is safe. The sirens remind dreamers and diarists alike that there is more to come, that silence for a few days guarantees nothing, that just surviving is the most that can be hoped for, is all that the word 'good' can mean. Maybe later, when everything is resolved one way or another—or, more likely, left unresolved but quietened down into an anxious stalemate—grieving will become possible and the past will be put in its place and futures will be able to unroll again. But right now, there is just this bombed city, this empty space or, as Anastasiia I. says, 'this hole, through which the wind sings and even rain drops' (March 22, p. 234). The temporality here is that of 'too soon'. It is not that the loss is denied—hence this is not a pathological state of melancholia—but grieving and mourning are blocked, emptying out the world.

Melancholia and loss are connected to trauma; trauma is, for Freud, linked ambiguously with the Death Drive. Trauma as the overflow of sensation that cannot be 'digested' through symbolic means is in some ways akin to the melancholic refusal or inability to work on grieving the lost object, but it goes further in externalising the source of the trouble. Trauma arises from outside, as an event that overwhelms the psyche. As described in the diaries and dreams, this incursion or invasion from the outside becomes concentrated in the sounds of the sirens that intrude all the time into psychic life, carrying with them not only the warning to take cover, which is their major function, but also all the harmonics of destruction. The noise of the sirens, freed from language and materialising as a 'wail', 'howl' or 'roar', are distress-filled articulations that have no semantic or symbolic content beyond signalling approaching trouble, but are experienced more for what they are in absolute, an acoustic atrocity that cannot be controlled. In the dreams and diaries, it seems as if the trauma of the Russian invasion becomes concentrated into this non-symbolic signal like a kind of psychotic object of the sort that Bion (1967) calls 'bizarre objects' – fragments of the mind that are disconnected from one another to protect the possibility of a modicum of sanity when the mind itself feels like it is under constant attack. The dreamers and diarists are not psychotic or paranoid: they really are under attack. But the traumatic sirens that persecute them through their evocation of the destructive power aimed at them are maddening in themselves, creating panic and filling up the mind with noise. As Oksana V. says, 'It seems to me that I will soon get used to this long-drawn roaring and that it will be my usual condition with a siren in my head' (March 11, p. 85). Perhaps this is what Lacanians mean by the Real: a traumatic kernel that cannot be reduced to a representation of something else.

In Freud's (1920/1955) formulation of trauma and destruction in *Beyond the Pleasure Principle*, the resurgence of traumatic material in dreams and symptoms, and famously in the play of his grandson, is linked with the question of why we might be drawn to repetition of events and experiences that are deeply distressing. Eventually, Freud declares this repetition to be an aspect of the Death Drive, the tendency to be found in all beings to seek a reduction of stimulation and hence to recede into nothingness. As this concept develops across Freud's thinking and into that of Melanie Klein, the Death Drive becomes more actively connected with destructiveness; in Klein's (1957/1975) case, the direct representation of the Death Drive in the mind is in unconscious feelings of envy. But this is later; in the immediate post-War moment, Freud is trying to understand the 'attraction' of suffering and deathliness, with destructiveness being an outcropping or 'projection' of this into the external world. As is often the case, it is worth attending to the description Freud gives of the 'fort-da' game played by his grandson Ernst to try to get some sense of what is being examined here. In this well-known story, the child is observed throwing a wooden reel into his curtained cot so that it disappears from view and then pulling it back out again, accompanying these actions with sounds interpreted as the German words 'fort' ('gone') and 'a joyful "da" ("there")' (Freud, 1920/1955, p. 15). Having been puzzled by the child's repeated act of throwing away his toys, Freud now realises that the game needs its two parts, the return as well as the eviction, and offers some reasonable interpretations of it, for instance that the boy is using it to master the difficult situation of separation from his mother or to express hostility towards her. However, as if dissatisfied with these fairly mundane explanations, Freud then introduces a deathly resonance into the material, pushing understanding of the child's quotidian play into metaphysical realms. In a footnote, Freud comments (p. 16n), 'When this child was five and three-quarters, his mother died. Now that she was really "gone" ("o-o-o"), the little boy showed no signs of grief. It is true that in the interval a second child had been born and had roused him to violent jealousy.' What is slightly strange about this is its *coolness* on the part of the child and of Freud. Perhaps the suggestion is that the premonitory 'mourning' carried out by the child in his game, added to by the Oedipal issues indexed by Freud (rivalry with the brother), has inured him to grief. However, as we know both from the history of the child Ernst (Benveniste, 2015) and from Peter Gay's (1988) biography of Freud, neither of them ever properly recovered from this death and instead there was for both a very deep and persisting melancholy, something that could not be recovered from fully, an unspoken haunting by the lost object, mother and daughter. O-o-o and a-a-a, fort and da, covers a lot of ground; here it is enough perhaps to say that it shows us a way both to face death and to seek refuge from it. Anastasiia B. writes on March 11:

> It's strange. Uncanny. Unheimlich. And all the rest of the words of this kind. I keep delaying the moment to rethink death. It's time, I think. I'm not trying to accept it, it's unreal. I'm talking about being able to think about it freely, as the brain (instinct of self-preservation) blocks everything connected to it. (p. 200)

In the dream and diary dreamscapes, there is plenty of this to and fro, this o-o-o and a-a-a. People join up to fight, volunteer to support others; they invoke patriotism and hatred, they find ways to confront as well as to flee their situation. They go out into the world and then retreat into the shelters; they show courage and they show fear. But the strongest connection is with what is left behind after the fort-da dynamic is gone and there remains only the sense of loss, that melancholic sense that death is pervasive and that something drives us towards it, whether we wish for it or not. *Beyond the Pleasure Principle* arises in part out of the recognition of the reality of traumatic dreams, in which the destructive legacy of fort-da is prominent. Many of the Ukrainian dreams have exactly this structure: whether they begin as comforting and idealised or not, they end with the trauma. Yelyzaveta B.'s dream from before the war of a Russian nuclear attack becomes in her mind a reality once the invasion starts: 'On March 15, my class coincided with the first air raid alarm in Lviv, and it was as if I was back in that dream without the opportunity to wake up. I had the desire to go blind and burst like a balloon' (recorded on March 28, p. 216). It is as if her inner life has pre-empted the war, yet when the war comes this precursive dream offers no protection. Stefaniia K. dreams of a 'totally black and smooth' drone that flies right up to her and 'protrudes a thing that can shoot' right in her face (March 23), whilst Ruta R. has an idyllic dream on April 05 of visiting an imaginary grandfather with her mother ('I guess my consciousness feeling the lack of happiness and good moments sends them to me in my dreams') only to be followed shortly afterwards by her 'worst dream' of the Russians coming and beating at her door with their rifle butts, followed by further dark dreams of violence and war (April 05, p. 75). It is not that these young women wish for death; it is rather that the motion of hope is swamped at this early point of the war by the overwhelming sensation of deathliness. The dreamscape as a destroyed landscape; what is thrown away does not come back whole.

Reparative Prospects

In this regard, looking for some comfort, it is worth mentioning one other psychoanalytic concept that grew out of the wars with which psychoanalysis had to deal: Melanie Klein's idea of the 'depressive position' (Klein, 1952). For Klein, this is partly to be understood as a phase of development that follows on from the 'paranoid-schizoid' period of earliest infancy, which is characterised by tendencies towards splitting and projection. However, the depressive position is better thought of as a way of experiencing and relating to oneself and the world (a 'position') that is sustained throughout life and is marked by a growing capacity to manage ambivalence and to feel both connectedness to others and guilt and responsibility towards them. The complexity of one's own impulses and the ambiguity of the external environment are both embroiled in structures of ambivalence: we have to learn to recognise that there is no purity, that everything is dappled, for better or worse, and that we can do damage to those we love. Living involves repeated disruption and repair. This perception links with an impulse towards 'reparation', which Klein (1955/1975, p. 133) defines as 'the variety of processes by which the ego feels it undoes harm done in phantasy, restores, preserves and revives objects.' Reparation allows the depressive position to be transcended, as children discover within themselves the resources to mitigate destructiveness, becoming more stable and also more psychologically realistic. This too follows through to adulthood as a hopeful indication of mature relationality, although we should note something else as well: the potentially punitive element of 'reparations' as demanded in many post-conflict settings and by many victims of oppression and abuse. That is to say, *reparation* may be an impulse towards making good; but if things have gone too far, if the destruction that has laid waste to a person or people is too great for forgiveness to be managed, then the campaign for *reparations* may be a call for what is perceived as *justice*, without which nothing can be reconciled or laid to rest. Without justice, the capacity to repair cannot be fully mobilised, resentments linger, the ghosts of past suffering continue to haunt, as has become ever clearer through the histories of recent conflicts and genocides and the failures as well as the successes of Truth and Reconciliation Commissions in different parts of the world (Frosh, 2019). Yet if justice is linked to reparations, it may be that reparation in the sense of merciful acknowledgment and healing, is still a long way off.

In the heat of the first few months of the Russian invasion, not to say a year and a half of continued war later, it looks unlikely that reparation, the rebuilding of a shattered world, can come about. The temporality of 'too soon' applies again here. It is too soon to fully register what is happening, too soon to predict the outcome, and certainly too soon for any rebuilding or indeed (a necessary component of the dynamic of reparation) to imagine forgiveness. 'Anger is eating me from inside', writes Yelyzaveta B. on March 02 (p. 213). For Anastasiia I. on March 09, the damage is both metaphorical and real:

> It seems I have cut veins on my arms, and I am bleeding all the time. So I go for a walk around the town, leaving a trail of drops after me; I drink tea while the blood from my veins drips on my knees; I hug the pillows, treacherously leaving inconspicuous spots on their backs. No one sees this blood; only I feel it. As if only I have these unhealed wounds. (p. 233)

Reparation has to be part of any healing process, but unhealed wounds and trails of blood do not allow for that; and in any case, reparation is required on the part of the aggressor and not the one who suffers violence. Psychoanalysis suggests that recognition and reparation will need to be the way forward if melancholia and trauma are to be overcome and some form of reconciliation is to be promoted, something other than deathliness achieved. There is not really any other way for war to come to an end, whether or not the fighting stops. Yet in this period, with the sirens still wailing and the blood still dripping, with anger, hatred, guilt and sadness prevailing, there seems little chance of that.

References

Benjamin, J. (1998). *Shadow of the other: Intersubjectivity and gender in psycho-analysis*. Routledge.

Benveniste, D. (2015). *The Interwoven lives of Sigmund, Anna and W. Ernest Freud*. The American Institute for Psychoanalysis.

Bion, W. (1967). *Second thoughts*. Heinemann.

Butler, J. (1997). *The psychic life of power*. Stanford University Press.

Butler, J. (2012). *Parting ways*. Columbia University Press.

Freud, S. (1957). Mourning and melancholia (J. Strachey, Trans.). In J. Strachey (Ed.), *The standard edition of the complete psychological works of Sigmund Freud, Volume XIV (1914-1916): On the history of the psycho-analytic movement, papers on metapsychology and other works* (pp. 237–258). Hogarth Press. (Original work published 1917).

Freud, S. (1955). Beyond the pleasure principle (C. J. M., Hubback, Trans.). In J. Strachey (Ed.), *The standard edition of the complete psychological works of*

Sigmund Freud, Volume XVIII (1920-1922): Beyond the pleasure principle, group psychology and other works, (pp. 1–64). Hogarth Press. (Original work published 1920).

Frosh, S. (1999). *The politics of psychoanalysis*. Palgrave-Macmillan.

Frosh, S. (2019). *Those who come after*. Palgrave.

Gay, P. (1988). *Freud: A life for our time*. Dent.

Klein, M. (1952). Some theoretical conclusions regarding the emotional life of the infant. In J. Riviere (Ed.), *Developments in psychoanalysis* (pp. 61–93). Hogarth Press.

Klein, M. (1975). The psychoanalytic play technique: Its history and significance. In M. Klein (Ed.), *Envy and gratitude and other works* (pp. 122–140). Delta. (Original work published 1955).

Klein, M. (1975). Envy and gratitude. In M. Klein (Ed.), *Envy and gratitude and other works* (pp. 176–235). Delta. (Original work published 1957).

Rose, J. (1996). *States of fantasy*. Clarendon Press.

Shapira, M. (2013). *The war inside*. Cambridge University Press.

Sharpe, C. (2016). *In the wake: On blackness and being*. Duke University Press.

Skelton, R. (2006). *The Edinburgh international encyclopaedia of psychoanalysis*. Edinburgh University Press.

5

'THE WORD REMAINS'[1]

War Diaries in Ruptured Time and Space

Magda Schmukalla

Me and my partner are in our kitchen, in our home in London. Our two children are upstairs in their room, watching their usual kids' series. I am preparing the batter for Polish pancakes, which I loved so much as a child, when suddenly we hear a high-pitched and extremely loud tone coming from my phone. For what feels like a long and intense second, I am disturbed and intuitively prepared for some extreme situation. But then a thought breaks through and draws me back to the reality of my Sunday afternoon: this siren is the test-alert about which I read in the papers this morning and about which people spoke on the market, when I bought apples for the pancakes. It is a test, a trial. It is not real![2]

I am relieved. I continue whisking the batter. My partner and I laugh nervously to thaw our bodies which froze for the second when the siren pierced through our everyday. It had freaked us out. While not linked to a real threat it still had brought into our life a material reminder of the possibility that an emergency or rupture could any time brutally change our life from one moment to another; disrupt our life to an extent that would go beyond a certain level of comprehension.

Since the 24th of February 2022, people in the whole of Ukraine have been living with the reality of air alerts. The piercing sound which announces potential or actual catastrophic emergencies has itself become part of the everyday. What for me felt and feels like the unimaginable exception, too extreme to be true, in Ukraine has become normality where bodies and minds live in a state of constant yet not always conscious alert. *Diaries of War and Life* documents the beginning of this shift towards the ordinariness of exceptions. The diaries are a compound archive of experiences, events and effects that characterised the first weeks of the full-scale war in Ukraine.

DOI: 10.4324/9781003449096-9

They contain descriptions of the shock, of loss, of fright, depression but also describe love, longing, and the importance of quotidian joy. Each of these descriptions, however, is marked by the presence and effects of a rupture or a catastrophic shift, the before and after the war.

This essay aims at acknowledging and tracing this experience of rupture through the words and word-arrangements that were captured in the diaries. More specifically, it aims to understand how the diaries trace the rupture that a war has torn into both material and psychic structures, which shaped everyday life in Ukraine before the war. In the last year, we have become used to seeing the destruction caused by the war through images of destroyed bodies or buildings, but what is less obvious is how a war destroys psychic arrangements. By showing how the ruination of external and cultural environments is deeply intertwined with internal experiences of collapse, this essay aims at better understanding the damage caused by a war to psychosocial forms of subjecthood, i.e. a form of subjecthood and experience which considers psychic and social-material processes as mutually constitutive and dialectically intertwined (Frosh, 2014; Frosh & Baraitser, 2008). It does so by tracing how a war destroys material and culturally symbolic structures that are necessary for experiencing life through coherent and shared parameters of time and space as well as by constructing an intersection between material-feminist understandings of physical void and a psychoanalytic understanding of the unconscious to theorise the non-temporal locus towards which being is catapulted when material and psychic structures are in ruins.

In times of war a society, I argue, slips towards the realm of unconscious being, which is a form of non-being that accumulates in the margins or cracks of what is consciously acknowledged as liveable and grievable life (Butler, 2016). The diaries, however, also show that such a rupture in psychosocial subjecthood does not automatically lead to chaos or despair, but rather to alternative arrangements of words and psychosocial matter, and with this to alternative arrangements of a collective subject. I call these alternative arrangements 'word remains' and attribute to them the radical creativity and criticality of feminine subjectivity.

Disrupted Time

'Last night I had my first panic attack in 7 days', writes Olha K. one week after the full-scale war broke out in Ukraine (March 2, p. 44). Like documented in many other diaries, she describes how the emotional response to the military attack arrived with a delay, as if the body needed more or a different kind of time to acknowledge a radical shift or rupture that had just taken place. In her description of the panic attack, she highlights the experience of losing a sense of time and orientation:

I realized that my memory erased all my movements from the previous week. i realized that I have been sleeping not in my apartment for 6 days now. why that? right, I had a plan to move from pokhyla's place to virmenska, to move out on February, 24, to stay there for a month, while vlad stays in portugal. where are the keys to the virmenska's place? who's in there now? i don't know. i gave the keys to ira kovalchuk, she hosted someone there. what else have I forgotten? how did it all even start? what plans did I have for the day? for the week? for next year? (Olha K., March 2)

Everyday life is usually configured of a multitude of practices and encounters each of which is in some relation to others. Commonly, we perceive the events of everyday life as either preceding or following or overlapping others, with this perception allowing for the experience and memory of a life that develops *in* time. Such flow of time places the presence between experiences of old and new, between past and future, and between young and old, experiences which create a sense of life as a movement. At times, however, this experience of a continuous flow is disrupted and time suspended, leading to, as Lisa Baraitser demonstrates, very different felt experiences of time—of 'time *not passing*', of time pooling or slowing down without end (Baraitser, 2017, p. 2).[3]

Diaries of War and Life documents how the full-scale war in Ukraine initiated such a suspension in time. While a before and after the beginning of the war can for many war chroniclers still be distinguished, the time of the 'after' turns into a blurred or fragmented mass in which daily life is no longer structured around the familiar flow of clock time, or of dates in the calendar and arrangements between friends, families, or institutions, but predominantly by irrupting news about survival or death of individuals and the rupturing sound of air alerts. Ihor K., whose diary records 79 air alarms in 55 diary entries, writes:

Air alarm 2:19–7:41 AM

The father of one of my students was killed at the training ground in Novoyavorivsk.

Mykola is alive. At the time of the bombing, he was already in another place. (…)

Alarm 7:55–8:41 AM. (March 14, p. 70)

While recurring patterns of micro-practices such as shopping, meeting friends, working, studying, taking a shower, or cooking usually fill days with meaning and form patterns around which a life as movement can be experienced, a war attacks any form of routinised arrangement or continuum. In doing so a war not only destroys bodies and buildings but also a sense of self and the self's positioning in time. It leaves a rupture in chronological time and plunges people into a threshold where time does not evolve in familiar periods and forms but feels unpredictable and unmemorable, leaving a gap at the centre of the self:

> I have been in a real mourning for the future, which will definitely never be the way I imagined [...] and for the past too, which will never be the way it seemed to go on forever. After all, they just shot my past and future down. And now I have to live with this emptiness in my chest. I have to live with this hole, through which the wind sings and even rain drops; sometimes crumbs of food and other trash fall there, but nothing can fill it anymore because the loss is too vast. It has hit me through. (Anastasiia I., March 22, p. 234)

What stands out in Anastasiia I.'s description of her experience of mourning is the materiality of an embodied gap that comes to the fore when chronological time as a continuity of past and future is destroyed. This means that chronological time is not only a cultural construct which shapes external, social matters but a structured entity or object which fills up the subject from within. When this entity or arrangement of chronological time, which is created and enacted through routinised actions and organised around shared and internalised calendars and clocks, is lost, as in the case of war, the subject is left with the experience of a hollowing out, an experience of unbecoming, in which the impression of being filled and solid is replaced by loss and the permeability of a void. Yet, what Anastasiia I.'s image also shows is that this void is not simply nothingness or absence but another space or locality which is ruled by unusual and uncanny sensations. While experienced as hollow it is not empty or static. Flows of air and matter pass through it yet seemingly nothing of meaning or durability can accumulate in the space that opens when time is shot down. Only crumbs of food and other trash fall there.

In actually or potentially attacking residential buildings, in displacing and separating families, and creating environments in which planning ahead or linking to previous actions or routines is made increasingly difficult (destruction of time) a war does not only destroy flesh and physical matter, but it also destroys the internal symbolic edifice of chronological time which in modern societies is a crucial paradigm for meaning making practices. But when destroying the meaning that is formed and held together by known pasts and futures the rupture caused by the war also reveals meaning's other, namely an experienced void or vacuum, which is life in its permeable and unpredictable form. A rupture in common signifying chains and practices makes this bare materialisation of life's other experienceable. It initiates felt encounters with life's energy prior to or beyond any structuring routines and contexts. Psychoanalytically speaking, it triggers encounters with unconscious or foreclosed formations of what is usually experienced as reality, moving subjects towards a so-called 'non-temporal locus', the unconscious, which according to Lacan is 'another locality, another space, another scene, the between perception and consciousness' (Lacan, 1998, p. 56).

Continuity and consistency within the perception-consciousness system means that what is perceived is experienced as in line with a systematically arranged experience of reality. A rupture in this system or symbolic contract, however, does not simply cause a gap in experience and knowledge of reality but brings to the fore what is opposite to what is perceivable, grievable and conscious, namely an unconscious non-temporal place—the consistently excluded. A place that is not structured according to the laws of chronological time or geographical space but is out of joint and yet sits at the centre of a person's embodied presence. A place where time pools or loops without rim, or as Ruta R. writes in her diary: 'Today it's been a month since the war began. A month has passed but February 25th hasn't yet come to me. Time has become too lengthy in the most awful way possible. Every day I've been living for a year, but February 25th isn't coming closer' (March 24, p. 74).

Disrupted Space

Like in the case of ordered and chronological time, a sense of ordered space makes individuals feel safe and alive (Ivinson & Renold, 2013, p. 371). Buildings and public places of a city are tied up with people's identities and images of themselves and others, but also with their most intimate feelings. The city space materialises cultural imaginations of a society's past and future, but it also forms an extended container with symbols and sites that remind a person or group of different events or phases in their life. Attacks on residential buildings and public sites during a war should therefore, as Robert Bevan argues, not be seen as collateral damage but as a strategic element of the violence used to weaken and, in some cases, systematically destroy a society, which usually finds it form and language in shared routines, laws and public infrastructures (Bevan, 2007).

The city space is thus not simply built of stone and mortar but also formed of and entangled with the language, signifying chains and affects that shape people's internal, psychic worlds and experiences. As such semiotic and aesthetic arrangement or text (Gottdiener & Logopoulos, 1986), the city is an extension of internal configurations of social subjecthood and embodied self. Its physical and aesthetic intactness and consistency are tightly interwoven with intact and consistent maps of a person's self while attacks on such external spaces coincide with traumatic ruptures in a culturally shaped subjectivity, potentially leading to extreme experiences of internal fragmentation.

On day eight of the war, Kateryna L. writes in her diary: 'Cities moan … Their moans stab my heart. Cities howl like real living things. Cities are also hurt. They bleed in smoke. They fall apart when missiles hit them' (March 3, p. 82). When a country is under attack, psychic pain does not have a defined place. It does not sit in some people while not in others. It is not an event of the individual mind but takes place at the threshold between internal and external worlds. For it is a pain that is triggered by the violent transgression of known boundaries between subjects and objects, between cities and soul. The pain felt when living under consistent threat of potential or actual attacks is felt as a pain that spreads across cities and landscapes. Objects turn into living beings suffering and expressing a pain that cannot be held while an internal sense of subjecthood and liveliness is being hollowed out, vacated:

> I've got an impression that I lose some part of myself every day. How can we rebuild a place where 100 people died? How can you visit a 'rebuilt' theatre if hundreds of people were buried alive in its basement? I imagined our Frankivsk theatre in Mariupol theater's place. People are hiding under our theatre as well, many people. And this building is like a living being. It's like a close person. You walk there, pass this building all your life, sit on its stairs, enter it to see a play, look at it, love it, every day. How is it possible? I have no energy left. I just feel how it gets harder to breathe. I feel like a little powerless human. My legs and arms are weak and constantly trembling even when I think I am standing calmly. (Anastasiia B., March 17, p. 202)

In times of war, the destruction of houses triggers a disturbance of psychic edifices with the reverberations of a bomb being felt beyond the geographical and physical scope of the detonating force. A building is no longer experienced as an external structure that is simply there to hold and organise independent individual lives or events, but physically and symbolically entangled with the presence and survival of life itself. Being intact it turns into an important material and symbolic defence against looming attacks. Yet when collapsing, this container of bodies as well as memories and hopes, tears down internal symbolic structures and destabilises meaning-making chains from within. The systematic occupation and annihilation of houses and public sites hence expels a person not only physically but also psychically from a known or familiar place inside a cultural and socio-historical context or continuum, catapulting them towards the state of a 'powerless human'—of a human who has been brutally ripped off their cultural shell and defences.

But again, those who survive military attacks physically experience this vacated material-cultural void, the internal/external scene of ruptured structures, not as simply empty but filled with rubble, corpses, and smoke, which are the physical and psychic relics of incomprehensible loss and violence and in excess of what can be acknowledged or processed—individually and collectively. The brutal destruction of buildings does therefore not only take away the presence of composed and stable entities and structures, it does not simply end societal being, but unleashes experienceable aspects of an incomprehensible and unbearable yet present other reality or matter. This other reality or void is, as the feminist-materialist theorist Karen Barad writes in relation to the quantum vacuum, not a nothingness or lack nor is it simply another entity or 'something', but a materially present and psychically experienceable state that is composed of the dynamism or energy of unstructured, trashed, or exploded psychosocial matter; which is matter prior or beyond any measurement or conscious symbolic, socio-cultural configuration—matter ripped off its holding context or frame. The psychosocial state unleashed through military attacks on familiar cultural environments hence frees the presence and experience of an 'unending dynamism' in which the psychic and social self is 'dispersed/diffracted through time and being' and with this in touch with its 'infinite alterity' (Barad, 2019, p. 531)—i.e. with a reality that is other to what a person and society is able to know if themselves—the unconscious, non-temporal locus, the consistently excluded.

Psychically, this means, I argue, that a society whose material and cultural edifices are under attack moves collectively closer towards the realm of the unconscious, which is the 'indefinable something' with no predictable or measureable compositions of time and space; a psychic site that is filled up with the matter of pre-ontic being and trauma and 'apprehended in its experience of rupture' only (Lacan, 1998, p. 56). A war, hence, initiates a shift from an ordered and recognisable, communicable form of being, psychically and socially *in* time and space, and towards an unmeasurable yet present void which usually is not seen or recognised in times when material or psychic amenities are not under attack.

Disintegration and Darkness

A subject who occupies a place in a spacetime continuum, a conscious subject, is always already caught up with its non-temporal, hollow, indefinable unconscious other. Yet, being brutally pushed towards the city's void or the psyche's unconsciousness unleashes painful experiences of loss and displacement, a loss of orientation and identity. With the temporal and spatial structures of an external environment being under attack also the scaffolding of internal structures (built of laws, memories, relationalities, identities) disintegrates, reviving a felt knowledge of the psyche's archaic state, i.e. of an embodied state before, during and close to birth, when no clear distinction between inside and outside, between self and other can yet be distinguished (Schmukalla, 2022). Psychoanalytically speaking, this state is a state prior to any recognition of loss or lost object, prior to any felt or feared castration by an external authority, and prior to a symbolic order which would allow for conscious, rational communication. For the modern subject an encounter with this pre-ontic subjectivity leads to extreme abject sensations of physical and mental unbecoming (Kristeva, 1987) or sensations of mental chaos and disintegration. Yelyzaveta B. who fled with her sister and her sister's partner to Poland writes:

> I can't recognize my reflection in the mirror at all. I've spent a long time, examining it; my reflection looks like a picture of an unknown girl in the Internet. I am frightened by how my ribs and shoulders are protruded. For the first time in my life, I think it's too much: I am too slim. What I look like is sharp corners, ribs, shoulders and elbows added by dark circles under my eyes. There are shades not only on my face but all over my body as if I myself were about to become a shade. I have become faded and darkened with nothing but eyes on my face: two jewels, also sharp and wicked. I want to hide away from my own looks but there is no place to hide away. (March 15, p. 215–216)

Describing the blurring and darkening of her known posture and look, Yelyzaveta B. captures the transition from a known, imaginary self towards an encounter with psychic life and the body in its unknown, blurred, unconscious formations where the boundaries to others, other bodies, other times, other places, disintegrate. Such drastic expulsion from a known, contextualised space and body drags the subject towards sensations of muteness and death:

> Now I noticed that everything I lived for, what I burned for, and what I aspired to before the war (...) left me and lost its meaning. And not only that, but life in general lost its meaning, so when I honestly asked myself: 'What's wrong with you?', I heard in response only: 'I think you just do not want to live. (Anastasiia I., April 6)

Where everyday routines and symbols arrange life into meaningful forms that can be lived in a shared and recognisable time-space continuum, a war destroys this continuum and pulls experience towards a non-verbal, supposedly meaningless state, associated with the indeterminable yet real possibility of sudden destruction and untimely death. Death is no longer something that has its place and time, attached to the end of an imaginary life path and away from youth but a possibility that could become reality and the end of it at any moment in and beyond time, not allowing for stark or fixed patterns or rhythms to occur. Constant yet unpredictable howls of sirens, missiles smashing buildings and bodies, destroyed city landscapes or news feeds documenting the many losses are inextricably interlinked with the destruction of psychic landscapes, unleashing the presence of an over-whelming destructive force which is turned against whatever is left. And this boundless fear of dying, the fading away of life as an embodied path of coherence and stability, also intrudes and shapes the moment of writing, expressed for instance in the fear of writing the last words in Khrystia M.'s diary:

> The situation is tense. For some reason, there were two sirens in a row. It is rare for Kalush. It's strange. Am I afraid? I'm afraid now. There's a heavy lump in my throat, like a stone. I can't move. I can't speak. Everyone near me in the bomb shelter is discussing the news. In Kyiv, a rocket just hit the area of the underground passage at the train station. I'm afraid. I am afraid that these words [...] I do not believe these words will be the last. But if [...] If so, I don't know. I want to cry. I feel cold all over my body. (March 2, p. 51)

Writing a war diary happens with a felt knowledge that words and this life could end at any time. Writing and speech, usually symbols and the mortar of life, turn into potential sites of destruction and death. Not only are buildings and bodies in danger of annihilation, but also the diary entry, the narrative, the possibility of arranging a life around beginnings and endings, is under threat.

A war kills bodies and destroys buildings. It traumatises particularly those who have lost a loved one and those who have lost their home. But a war also attacks on an internal, psychic level. For in rupturing culturally configured and trans-generationally shared arrangements of time and space, a war also causes, as traced in the words of the war chroniclers, internal damage and displacement. Here 'internal displacement' does not refer to those refugees who had to leave their physical homes while remaining within their country's borders, but to everyone who experiences a psychic form of displacement or rupture in material-discursive and emotional arrangements which are crucial for forming a coherent and communicable experience of self and interpersonal relationships. 'I'm not fighting at the frontline', writes Bohdan S. (March 25, p. 239), 'but I'm already dying [...]'.

Remains

For those who must cope with such experiences of internal displacement, a turn towards a collective, national identity and unity is often a life-saving psychic mechanism and form of resistance. Another path towards preserving a coherent self and sense of continuity is, as evidenced in many diary entries, the enactment of symbolic everyday routines and encounters such as cooking, planting, drinking coffee, or making love. 'I love everyone', writes Olha K., one day before acknowledging her first panic attack. 'Everyone who writes about being alive, everyone who helps, everyone who does something, hugs, calms down, sends music, news, cooks to eat, strokes a cat, goes to the pharmacy, takes photos, or saves lives' (March 1, p. 43). Each of these micro-practices becomes a sustaining action against incommensurable destruction and despair—a protection against the void that opens around the gaps torn into external and internal structures. But there is, I argue, yet another mechanism of human survival, a form in which life continues against the odds of a suspended time and destroyed space, that can be observed in the diary project. This other form of survival and resistance, I argue, is the act of writing about the war and rupture in words that remain close to the void and unconscious alterity of the self, which means in words that are formed without there being a narrator's self who could master the narrative; i.e. a form of writing that persists even if there is no story to tell nor a composed protagonist who walks through time and space from beginnings to endings.

What can be known, said, and lived in a state in which the time-space continuum and kinship relationships are transindividually and transgenerationally disturbed? How does life happen and flow if the contours of time, space and relational orders have been attacked and blurred? Do speech and subjectivity survive such a rupture and if so how? The texts in *Diaries of War and Life* offer answers to these questions. They demonstrate how experiences of body, of subjectivity, and kinship bonds persist even when a known or familiar connection to order and symbolic arrangements is lost. Being continues but shifts towards the reality of the void or gap that emerges when conscious images and ideas of who 'I' or 'we' are incapacitated or ruptured. A sudden encounter with this hollow place that is vacant of the usual structures and edifices triggers sensations of powerlessness and disorientation. Yet, while no longer 'something' or 'someone' the matter and psychic life of the void or the unconscious is also not nothing, but rather, as Barad puts it, 'a desiring orientation toward being/becoming, innumerable imaginings of what might yet be/have been' (Barad, 2019, p. 529). Or to put it in psychoanalytic words, losing the self yet continuing to be[4] means moving close to life in its desiring, demanding, unrealised, or unrecognised form, or closer to life in its unconscious formations as the 'something other (that) demands to be realized' (Lacan, 1998, p. 25).

In the realm of the void or unconscious being, thinking goes on but is untied from the usual symbols and frames, the usual points or figures of orientation. In such a situation, words, written or uttered, I argue, are remains or remainders of desired pasts or futures, of times yet to be realised and imagined, times that yet 'be/have been', and that are placed close to the gap that opens up when conscious and familiar arrangements of time and space are brutally disturbed. Such 'word remains' do not communicate the state of being, they are not part of an ontology nor expressed within the law and language of the historical subject, a subject experiencing and moving along the path of history, but these 'word remains' spring from an embodied vibrating, desiring force which pushes a voice into being in moments when life and death cannot be told apart. Such words are close to the indeterminable yet present energy of the void or unconscious, where relations and laws sit in unknowable and uncontrollable forms, and the subject emerges not as a separate, speaking entity, but in gestures towards desired, not yet realised forms of subjectivity or community.

'Word remains' turn the suffering caused by the trauma of the rupture into 'rhythms, signs, forms' (Kristeva, 1987, p. 8) and as such witness the crisis of structure and closeness to the void. These word creations are not spoken from within the realm of the law or narrative. They are uttered without knowing beginnings or ends, without knowing the terms of punishment or reward. They are words that cannot be mastered for they rise directly from, or are close to, the gaps torn into the realm of mastery and knowledge.

'Word remains' spoken from or close to the unconscious are further not words that can be used to work through wounds. They are not words through which justice can be restored, for they are themselves structured by the reality of the wound or gap (Schmukalla, 2022). In fact, many of the words captured in the diaries are often aggressive, envious, or at times nationalist, forming images of violent forms of revenge against Russians, but being uttered in the precarious form of a war diary, they also always are vulnerable, interrupted, incoherent, irritated, unstable, unpolished, or hushed. As words they are under the same threat as the buildings and bodies of a city under attack, and as such they moan and bleed. They acknowledge the moment of unpredictable endings and yet continue to arrange letters. They push against a state of felt lawlessness or injustice not by imposing a different or old law, not by pretending unity where there is disintegration, but by surviving the attack's muting and humiliating force and by doing so uttering a forceful desire for change and being.

Such words, I argue, belong to the non-ontic state that concerns ethics not ontology. Or using the imagery of a Greek war myth, they are the words uttered from the position of Antigone, not Creon; a position that is not determined by culturally established laws and borders, but by an embodied knowledge of felt kinship and interpersonal dependency and with this by the knowledge of the pain that is caused by indeterminable and violent transgressions outside the law. Such words then do not utter what being or life means or how it could be organised, but are a reminder of life's precariousness, its formation prior to becoming and recognition. Words uttered close to the incommensurable yet present void, which is not nothing, nor something, but a form of being that utterly challenges the being we know and are able to control. Being able to continue writing or uttering words in this state means speaking from the site of a desiring, unrealised civilisation, which speaks beyond the means and concepts of the war: 'I don't attack you', writes Kristeva in relation to poetic language which is formed close to experiences of the abject, 'I speak (or write) my fear or my pain. My suffering is the lining of my word, of my civilization' (Kristeva, 1987, p. 14).

When concluding her autoethnographic analysis of the transgenerational inheritance of the Korean war, ethnographer Clara Han points to the gendered dynamics that were at play when confronting the legacy of the war. Han observes how naming the inherited violence and the desire for sustaining 'relatedness against and despite the corrosion of war and displacement' (Han, 2020, p. 154) was a task that had been taken over almost entirely by the girls and women of the family. She argues that in the wake of war kinship, community, and, I would like to add, subjectivity cannot be attained by claiming 'mastery over a narrative as in the contest between fathers and sons' (p. 154)—this path of human inheritance is as if blocked by the ravaged internal structures that the war has left behind. Instead, relational life and subjectivity have to be formed in or close to the archaic region of the feminine or maternal, where words are present yet without fixed meaning; where life exists not in paths but in cycles and rhythms as well as 'through attention to the small, the diminutive, the low' (p. 154)—the domestic everyday. It is in this convoluted and unruly everyday that feminine structures and forms of subjectivity and communication are present and needed. Structures that as psychoanalyst and artist Bracha Ettinger argues are formed in closeness to a felt knowledge of the ab/presence of the m/Other, so close to intrauterine experiences of entangled part-bodies and the non-ontic yet real state of the subject's absence (Ettinger, 2006). It is not that this is a place where thinking and words are not present. Yet thinking and words function differently, leading to unexpected and vulnerable words and thoughts which are formed in close awareness of life's precariousness and pain.

'I finally started writing a diary, together with the students. We created a chat in Telegram yesterday and now there are 44 participants, although they are mostly girls', writes Bohdan S. (March 3, p. 237). So, when looking at *Diaries of War and Life* I wonder whether the task of writing a diary, of archiving and speaking beyond the collapse of external and internal structures, of collecting and preserving the crumbs, the rubble, the corpses that occupy the void, where known communication and laws have been replaced by brutal force, can be seen as a deeply feminine form of resistance. Feminine not in the sense that it is restricted to 'girls' but a task that requires a desiring subject, a subject 'that might yet be/have been' and thus a subject which is able to speak without having to conquer and control the narrative or the place of a father or law.

'All that remains is a broken window, a broken cobblestone, a broken life', writes Viktoria Y. at the very end of her diary (March 5, p. 84). The end of her diary also forms the end of a cycle during which I read 24 of the translated diaries, with each diary ending abruptly, leaving me with no knowledge of the writer's whereabouts and wellbeing, and hence with an experienced trace of the rupture described by the chroniclers. At the same time, the end of each diary would also move me to the next diary and with this back to the beginning of the war, throwing my imagination and thought, again and again, back to the 24th of February 2022, to the beginning of the war that still has no end. In reading the chroniclers' words that were written close to the void or abyss that the war had torn open therefore meant that reminders of the reality and truth of the war, which I had felt so strongly in February and March last year but since had repressed, had re-entered my life. As such these war diaries stand as 'word remains' or as living monuments of an ongoing catastrophe, whose truth can only be known by those who remain close to life's unknowable and indeterminable other, i.e. close to a feminine, unconscious knowledge of life's unpredictable yet present and desiring dynamism and energy:

The word remains

And in someone unchanging remains – muteness.

The truth stands, shelled and still on guard.

And the sun will remain, no matter what the card turns out. (Victoria Y., March 5, p. 84)

Notes

1 Viktoria Y. (March 5, p. 84). Emphasis added.
2 Test-alert message was sent by the British government to all citizens in the UK on Sunday 24th of April, at 3 pm ... the actual alert was triggered at 2:59 pm.
3 Emphasis in the original.
4 'Even if I lose myself, I am' (Lacan, 1966, p. 136).

References

Barad, K. (2019). After the end of the world: Entangled nuclear colonialisms, matters of force, and the material force of justice. *Theory & Event, 22*(3), 524–550.

Baraitser, L., (2017). *Enduring time*. Bloomsbury Publishing.

Bevan, R. (2007). *The destruction of memory: Architecture at war*. Reaktion Books.

Butler, J. (2016). *Frames of war: When is life grievable?*. Verso Books.

Ettinger, B. (2006). *The matrixial borderspace* (Vol. 28). University of Minnesota Press.

Frosh, S. (2014). The nature of the psychosocial: Debates from studies in the psychosocial. *Journal of Psycho-Social Studies Volume, 8*(1), 159–169.

Frosh, S. & Baraitser, L. (2008). Psychoanalysis and psychosocial studies. *Psychoanalysis, Culture & Society, 13*, 346–365.

Gottdiener, M. & Lagopoulos, A.P. (Eds.). (1986). *The city and the sign: An introduction to urban semiotics*. Columbia University Press.

Han, C. (2020). *Seeing like a child: Inheriting the Korean War*. Fordham University Press.

Ivinson, G. & Renold, E. (2013). Subjectivity, affect and place: Thinking with Deleuze and Guattari's Body without Organs to explore a young girl's becomings in a post-industrial locale. *Subjectivity, 6*(4), 369–390.

Kristeva, J. (1987). On the melancholic imaginary. *New Formations, Number 3*, 5–18.

Lacan, J. (1998). *The four fundamental concepts of psychoanalysis: The seminar of Jacques Lacan, Book XI (A. Sheridan, Trans., J.-A. Miller, Ed.)*. Norton.

Schmukalla, M. (2022). Memory as a wound in words: On trans-generational trauma, ethical memory and artistic speech. *Feminist Theory*. Advance online publication. 10.1177/14647001221119993.

6

THE IMAGE IN RUINS

Martta Heikkilä

Is there anything that unites a sunflower, a tree cut off from its roots and a human heart? The war in Ukraine, and the reports and recorded footage of this event, has compelled people to unburden and process their experiences of it through other pictorial representations, such as drawing and painting. In this article, I wish to examine themes aroused by the war as reflected in a selection of images made by Ukrainian university students. The approach to my analysis is provided by Jacques Derrida's idea of ruins—both with respect to his notion of the image that is always already scattered and never complete, as well as in drawings as images of ruins, of ruined futures.

The images appear as documents from the early days of the war, a period from February to May 2022. At that time, no one knew what the military invasion would bring with it over the coming months or even years. At the time of writing this article, in early 2023, the war continues, with no end in sight.

In this sense, the images may be observed as kinds of events: they document what is happening at a particular historical moment in Europe and, concurrently, are seen from highly personal viewpoints. The interest in these images lies primarily in their sense of witnessing and expressing the violence of the war.

Flowers

The common sunflower (Helianthus annuus),[1] or soniashnyk in Ukrainian, has grown on the central and eastern steppes of Ukraine since the middle of the eighteenth century. It is the national flower of Ukraine, and until the Russian invasion, Ukraine was the world's largest exporter of sunflower

DOI: 10.4324/9781003449096-10

seeds and oil. Recently, the sunflower has become an even more important symbol of the country.

Since the beginning of the war in 2022, many people have sent sunflower seeds to Russian embassies or laid sunflowers outside of them in different parts of the world as a show of silent protest and solidarity for Ukrainians (Wulfeck, 2022). The idea of the sunflower as the symbol of peace is not new, however. In the 1990s, a vast field of sunflower seedlings was planted at a Ukrainian missile base. As a consequence of the dissolution of the Soviet Union Ukraine inherited a large number of nuclear weapons. After having been given international security assurances, Ukraine gave up these weapons, and the planting of sunflowers marked the completion of the disarmament process.

In the drawings of sunflowers made in the midst of the war, the sunny tones of yellow have given way to another tonal hue—that of rust. The vitality of the flowers has turned into a more fragile, almost bloodstained representation: sunflowers coloured by red hands and bloody feet in Uliana Pasternak's pastel drawings (Image 6.20, p. 158), or a bleeding flower surrounded by black carnivorous plants, as suggested by Eva Alvor (Image 6.2, p. 143). While the symbolism of these different hues in the blossoms is evident, the emotional charge of the images is heightened. The plant that up until the war brought prosperity to the country and provided a distinctive image of the national sentiment, now resembles a fragile, wrecked simulacrum of itself, a withered memory of the flower, a symbol of a damaged nation.

Ruins

Looking at an image of a flower offers various interpretations. Should we consider it a realistic imitation of a botanical species, a familiar symbol of a nation, or rather as a sign of indescribable ravage and of personal loss, a ruin that appears as a trace left by the war in Ukraine?

According to the philosopher Jacques Derrida, ruins are at the foundation of every image. In *Memoirs of the Blind: The Self-Portrait and Other Ruins* (1991/1993), he suggests that we can never grasp the image in the fullness of its meaning. The reason for this fundamental deficiency is ontological: an image presents itself to us, not so much in what we observe, but conversely, as if through what we do not see. We may see images only because we fail to perceive their presence in their entirety. With this seemingly paradoxical claim, Derrida proposes that in an image there is always an invisible, 'spectral' absence in what we see. Instead, we perceive as if we were looking past the images. Their meanings may be caught only indirectly, by means of remembering, associations and thinking. What Derrida calls 'ruins' announces a loss of integrity that structures the image.

According to this deconstructionist notion, the image is ontologically never simply present to us. While it shows itself, the image never presents a totality of sense. Therefore, it remains 'workless' (*désœuvrée*). As a result, it remains beyond our categories of knowledge: the meaning of the image is not to be reduced to any single message nor is it to be captured only through means of concepts.

In his critique of the dominance and primacy of seeing, Derrida's notion of art and visibility contrasts with the concept of *phainesthai*, 'to appear'. In Plato's *Republic*, the *phainesthai* relates to the notion of truth. It refers to visibility that arises from the ontological 'appearances' of things. Appearances emerge from visibility, which makes them deceptive, in contrast to the truth that is apprehended by the intellect (Plato, 1997, 479B–480A, 509D–510A, 532C1, 532C7–8). The *phainesthai* therefore opens the way to phenomena or perceived objects, facts and occurrences. Despite its doubtful implications in Plato's metaphysics, Derrida argues that the spectral, hallucinatory 'believing to see' and, at the same time, the predominance of *eidos*—'idea' or 'form'—has regulated theories of art from Plato to Edmund Husserl (Derrida, 1996/2010, p. 4). According to them, the image would allow us to see the objective ideality. By this, Derrida points to the notion that the object and the meaning of the image would be attainable by reason via perception, thus appearing separable from its materiality and the influence of different contexts.

The threat from outside is embodied by missiles. During the war, Russia has repeatedly launched waves of missiles and drone attacks on different parts of Ukraine. Among the heaviest of them was in November 2022, when more than a hundred missiles targeted several cities and districts along with the essential energy infrastructure (Foltynova, 2022). Until that time, Ukraine had used mostly Soviet-era defence systems, but as the year 2022 progressed, Western countries have been pressed to send more modern devices to Ukraine.

In one of the drawings, a woman with braided hair and without eyes is holding a missile in her hands, while in a drawing by Anastasiia B., another weapon spouting fire is heading towards the ground (Image 6.4, p. 144). In a more stylised image by Ihor Kolesnyk, a blue-faced man is threatened by missiles surrounding him (Image 6.14, p. 154). In the latter two pictures the black, empty background is striking. In the drawing by Anastasiia B., the darkness is impenetrable, whereas in Ihor Kolesnyk's, the background is structured by angular constructions hiding the missiles. In these images, there is a sense of panic and uncertainty: do we know who the enemy is?

According to Derrida, drawing is not based on perceiving clear-cut forms, but on the idea that perception is always conditioned by blindness and ruins. In drawing, we never see the drawn thing itself, but only what lies beyond the traits (1991/1993, pp. 55–56).[2] This means that the visible elements of the image, the lines and the traces, do not depict anything that already exists in the world. In lieu of representing and reproducing available forms, drawing forms *itself* in the act of drawing and in front of the spectator's look. In drawing, lines produce other lines and traces by making space for them. On the ground of an incompleteness that is in ruins and on the verge of falling apart before our eyes, the viewer constructs an image that is always in a fleeting, nascent state.

What does Derrida argue by saying that art exists in ruins? 'Ruins' are a metaphor for remains—what is left undone, in a state of decay and destruction. Ruins are the remains of disintegration, but they are also a sign of the incompleteness of destruction: of what has endured or survived. After a thing is destroyed, its ruins remain as fragments and traces of what has been. With the expression of ruins, Derrida suggests that the meaning of the image is never completely within the reach of the spectator. Art always already exists in ruins in our eyes, to the extent that it is defined by what Derrida calls the *rien à voir*, which is a double entendre. By it, he refers to both blindness in art—there is 'nothing to see' in it, as we can perceive only details of the image, hence its remains and never the whole image at once—and to the issue that art means a lack of relation: art has 'nothing to do with' writing and speaking of it (Derrida, 1991/2021, p. 99). The attempt to understand what the image 'means' would imply simply grasping the unvaried, full and original 'inner meaning' that would correspond with the image's content, even if it were expressed in different external variations (Derrida, 1978/1987, p. 22).[3] An attempt to make total sense of the image, however, proves to be impossible: in its details, traits and traces, an image is too multifaceted to be apprehended in totality, and it always leaves more space for interpretation than a single reading can achieve. Instead, he argues, something in the image will always remain unknown to us. By suggesting that the meaning of the image is scattered from the beginning, Derrida aims to reach beyond the traditional hierarchy of form and content, stating that the two never fully coincide in a work of art.

The image now shows itself only by first being disassembled. Only by supplementing it may the spectator approach the ruins of vision. In Derrida's hands, the traditional Modernist idea of the coherence of the image in which the image and its intended meaning integrate into a whole, appears to be an illusion. Instead, the spectator is faced with mere ruins—traces and traits—on which the possible sense of the image must be constructed. The process calls forth not only what we see, but the realms of thinking and memory alike.

Stillness and anxiety prevail in the images of shelters. For someone who has not experienced the war, to look at images of the places where people sought protection is especially distressing. In those pictures, the symbolic level of representation ceases to exist as one sees the depictions of shelters, similarly to those shown on television and in the newspapers. One of the most accurate examples of this are Marharita Zavhorodnia's black-and-white drawings, made in almost documentary style (Image 6.22, p. 160; Image 6.23, p. 161). She depicts deserted rooms with bunk beds and mattresses without anyone sleeping on them. Nightfall is seen between the curtains. These scenes reveal a need for withdrawal from the world in the midst of chaos. Along with fear, the loss of comfort, privacy and personal space are almost unimaginable to someone who has not lived through a war.

It is obvious that neither visual nor linguistic means suffice to make complete sense of the image, which suggests nothing but the difference between the appearance and disappearance of the depicted thing (Derrida, 1991/1993, p. 55). Such a notion concerning the image's disintegration and transience resonates with Derrida's thinking about language, his most important philosophical point of reference. In language, he argues, the spoken word is heard and understood, but nothing in speech will make a word visible. Indeed, the absence and withdrawal of the thing are at the core of emerging meanings in both image and language alike; language arises from what is not said, whereas images emerge between their invisible, ghostly traces, the image in ruins (Derrida, 1991/1993, pp. 2–3).

The image is not the endpoint of seeing, but rather seeing begins from the image. Yet, everything is there, on the surface of the image.

The Human Figure: Between Good and Evil

The drawings of human figures display a sense of disintegration which occurs from the outside, causing the human body to fall apart. The images suggest that this may happen in two ways, either under external physical pressure, or when the source of affliction is more internal, born inside the human figure carrying a burden (Anastasiia B., Image 6.5, p. 145). Evil assumes several figures, most distinctively that of the devil.

Emaciation has made the look startlingly empty in the face of a Buddha-like figure in Ihor Kolesnyk's watercolour (Image 6.15, p. 154). The petrified legless man is depicted in a sitting pose, whose shape is little more than that of a skeleton. A retreat from reality implies passivity: the serenity of the Buddha can be seen like that of the living dead. Mutilation, a state that may never again lead to integrity, is visible in two other watercolours, one by Kolesnyk (Image 6.16, p. 155) and one by Anastasiia B. (Image 6.6, p. 146). Here, human figures are presented concretely in ruins—body parts blowing apart, as if destroyed by an explosive force. The theme of disjecta membra, remaining scattered fragments, is repeated in violent images of hearts torn apart—romantic symbols for the site of emotions and the organ that belongs to each one of us, forming what is innermost to us.[4] The fragments of bodies, like archaeological remains, are of solid quality, however. The heart is the core of the self. The heart is mine singularly, but this singularity is common to everyone. To rip the heart apart is to destroy the person to whom it belongs.[5]

What is the role of the devil? Is it a reaction to the events of war? Is the devil the Russian leader and army? Is the devil inside of everyone?

In myths and art, the devil has assumed forms such as demons, evil spirits, Lucifer, Faust, to name just a few.[6] Devils are often presented as conventional figures, part animal and part man, with wings, tail, snout, claws and horns. The Devil, the personification of evil, puts humans to the test: how much will they resist pressure?

According to the common Christian idea, evil is located in sensual urges that are considered morally reprehensible. In his *Religion within the Bounds of Bare Reason* (1793–1794/2009, esp. 6:32–39), Immanuel Kant suggests, however, that evil must not be sensual and instinctive but intelligible, so that it can comprehend morality but also consciously reject it. Like good, evil refers to actions that human beings rationally choose to do, and we adopt freely good and evil maxims. Both good and evil are therefore objects of moral reason. To accentuate a human being's propensity to evil, Kant introduces the concept of 'radical evil', the belief that human beings have a natural tendency to be evil.[7] Radical evil refers to a conscious and deliberate will to act against the universal moral law, which Kant also calls the categorical imperative: 'Act only according to that maxim whereby you can, at the same time, will that it should become a universal law' (1785/1993, p. 30). According to this principle, a human action is only morally good if it is done from a sense of duty.

In Kant, radical evil, or action against the moral law, means the universal possibility of moral evil, as laid out in *Religion within the Bounds of Bare Reason* (1793–1794/2009). It implies that a human being may either freely obey or not obey the duties of the categorical imperative, commanded by reason, which is the source of all obligations. Radical evil offers subjective, unconditional grounds for evaluating motivations for action: an action is morally good if it follows from mere respect towards the law. Otherwise, action that derives from profit or any kind of extrinsic motivation, such as sensual attraction, means disobedience to the criteria of the categorical imperative.

According to Kant, by using one's reason, one can choose either good or evil. Our possibilities for both are equal; both good and evil are human qualities.

While missiles are weapons that bring concrete destruction, another recurring symbolic element is more metaphorical, although no less obvious in the context of the war: the devil. The devil is a familiar personification of evil: a destructive force that in various shapes—Satan, goat, dragon, serpent, fallen angel—appears across different cultures, religions and times. In a striking drawing by Anastasiia B., a horned, impersonal figure painted in dark hues of watercolour appears to 'save' a naked, faceless woman (Image 6.7, p. 147). Is the depicted woman not able to recognise the deception by the figure, ostensibly a saviour in disguise, such that she cannot see the devil's true nature? Or is her blindness a condition that is typical of a traumatic situation, where it can be unclear who is seeking refuge and who is in the position of offering shelter? In other drawings by Anastasiia B. (Image 6.8, p. 148; Image 6.9, p. 150), two devil-like characters are climbing on a plant that resembles a tree and a horned, blue-haired female is pictured on the centre of a flag with a yellow cross.

The faces of evil, often embodied by the image of the devil, convey an idea of horror in several drawings. First, the spectator encounters the gaze and the eyes of the human faces. If, to borrow a familiar cliché, 'the eyes are the mirror of the soul', what do they see in these images?[8] Do they perceive massacres and other war crimes happening, as in the drawings by Ihor Kolesnyk? In these works, frantic, screaming faces, recalling Edvard Munch's painting *The Scream* (1893), fill the space. Munch's Expressionist painting reveals a deep feeling of anxiety, although by looking at the painting we cannot tell what has provoked the scream. In both Munch's *Scream* and Kolesnyk's drawings (Image 6.17, p. 155), indescribable emotions seem to leave nothing but an eruption of energy, a material trace of a power the spectator can only imagine. It can be either the feeling of horror emerging from inside the figure, or a scene of horrors before one's eyes, or both.

However, it is also possible to interpret the devil as a catalyst, not necessarily only for evil, as in the novel *The Master and Margarita* (1928–1940), by Mikhail Bulgakov. By showing man's idea of the unrighteous, its awareness can be constructive and even lead to good activities in the future.

Sites of Trauma

The most tangible ruins are probably those of buildings that have now become derelict. Since the earliest days of the war in Ukraine, we have seen media images of bombed houses and the victims of attack standing by the ruins of buildings and in homes that have been razed to the ground, people forced to stay in cellars and temporary shelters.

Together with food, water, clothing and sleep, shelter is a necessity for anyone's physiological survival.[9] While Anastasiia B.'s watercolour and ink drawings display the devastation of a city where houses are burning (Image 6.10, p. 150), Ihor Kolesnyk (Image 6.18, p. 156) and Uliana Pasternak (Image 6.21, p. 159) turn their gaze upon more restricted, allegorical spaces of stillness and withdrawal. In their drawings, bent-over human figures are seeking refuge in a house or a suitcase. Cramped quarters seem to afford more safety than larger spaces, as the proximity of the walls limits the space, and the presence of other people may ward off unwanted persons and threats.

The struggle to lead a life among ruins means seeking protection against inhuman conditions as well as encountering an unknown future in which the perspective of time does not exist as it did before. In such living conditions, the prospects of a meaningful future may be coloured by trauma. Instead of building a life from the ruins, trauma can present an obstacle to this process. In the psychological framework, trauma means damage to the mind that occurs because of a distressing event. It is often the result of an excessive amount of stress that exceeds one's ability to integrate the emotions involved in that experience.

However, from a more philosophical viewpoint, trauma may not be only an injury, but an ontological state: it points to the fact of being exposed to the world that conditions our ways of being and knowing. In this sense, trauma might not be only a 'disorder' in a negative sense, a state out of the ordinary, but our state of existence that is affected by a plethora of things surrounding us. Our life is filled with the unexpected, unknown, and what cannot be assimilated, both good and bad, that come back to us, haunts us, even. In our minds, such experiences result in memories, images, thoughts, flashbacks and dreams. They mark a temporality of experiences and have a force to change our relation to ourselves and others.

Screaming and other kinds of expression of horror can be devastating. Apathy, the suppression of senses and feelings, can be a consequence of situations in which stress and anxiety are overwhelming. Such apathy often results from witnessing horrific acts, such as killing and violence in war, incidents that may lead to post-traumatic stress disorder (Bisson et al., 2015). Insensibility has left ruined faces behind faces that are no longer able to see, they refuse to look around them, or may only cast their eyes inwards; what is there to see, have they already seen everything? The faces that appear in an image by Anastasiia B. are black, which makes them look blank and hollow (Image 6.11, p. 151), or the eyes have been torn away and displaced, perhaps in front of scenes they would never have wanted to see (Image 6.12, p. 152). We must behold the images as if we saw past their remains. This is necessary to understand what it means to see the world as meaningful again. To cover one's eyes with hands marks a voluntary act and a choice when facing distress and terror (Luzganova, Image 6.19, p. 157; Alvor, Image 6.1, p. 143). Carrying an unnamed burden means taking a weight on one's shoulders—a weight that hangs as if it were a cloud, black or grey. How can one bear such a burden without collapsing under its stifling weight? The unspeakable load makes one turn the eyes downwards, away from the sight (Anastasiia B., Image 6.13, p. 153).

Meera Atkinson's concept of 'traumatic writing' is defined as 'an attempt to liberate the unconscious and speak of the unspeakable and the literally unthinkable' (Atkinson, 2013, p. 248). The central theoretical question in Atkinson's analysis concerns the possibility to bring the trauma to language. As a psychological symptom, trauma generally resists language, but to what degree it does so, is not clear: is trauma beyond words, as it is for psychoanalysts, or entirely unthinkable, as Derrida suggests in *The Specters of Marx* (1993/1994, pp. xix–xx)? According to Derrida's argument, we lack the language to approach trauma. Yet, poetic language can, by its effects, convey an experience reminiscent of the experience of trauma in that its meaning is never available as such.

A relevant question here is, to what degree is trauma present, and can it be articulated in the first place? For Derrida (1993/1994, p. xix), trauma remains distant because it is outside of time: it is like a ghost in that it no longer belongs to time—only its *effect* can be felt in time.[10] In this sense, trauma comes close to Derrida's concepts of ruins and trace: they are signs of absence that we encounter in the present which cannot be expressed by words. Trauma remains strange, but it still addresses the living like a spectre, being neither dead nor alive, neither presence nor absence, but other.

If anything like Atkinson's 'traumatic writing', a poetic approach to trauma, is possible, the images from Ukraine make us inquire whether traumatic *drawing* could be made. Images that, without saying a thing or by saying it ambiguously, are ruins of experiences themselves: traces that are only partial presentations. They evoke lived traumas, simultaneously singular and shared, by witnessing the events. In this way, the drawings discussed above work as mediums of the unspeakable and even of the unthinkable, which allow them a temporality of their own: time of the ghost, not always visible but still present, impossible to remember but unforgettable. The traumatic memories not only resemble, but even are ruins themselves.

What will the ruins allow us to see? Does Derrida's idea of the images in ruins destroy the possibility of showing something, or are the ruins rather a condition for seeing? His theory of ruins reminds us of the fact that the image is never solely in the hands of its maker, but the spectator's duty is to collect the ruins together and make them meaningful in the very moment of reception. Images in ruins proliferate in the minds of receivers and give birth to new, different images. Is it the same as Theodor Adorno's frequently cited statement about the possibility of creating art after the horrors of war—'To write poetry after Auschwitz is barbaric' (Adorno, 1951/1967, p. 34)? This claim probably refers to the failure of words after events that have produced a radical break between past things and what is said about them, between what has happened and our means of communicating that. This chasm makes us ask whether the addressee will ever succeed in grasping the message (Nosthoff, 2014).[11] How to define the position of art after

Ukraine and many other ongoing conflicts? When will the time for the 'after' arrive?

Contrary to Hegel, for Derrida art is far from 'a thing of the past'. Art's possibility of showing things, as well as its possibility to exist, must be sought *in* ruins which, however, remain like fragments, in contrast to destruction. Instead, we can no longer have the illusion of attaining any kind of permanent state of peace or of achieving shared harmonious images of a world without contradictions. The image itself is never total in that it is subject to conflicting, inconsistent interpretations, even unsolvable differends.[12] The image always leaves things ambiguous and under suspicion, as words will fail to convey fully the experience of Ukraine at war. The idea that presentations have already failed in what they reveal perhaps means abandoning the idea that experiences might be shared without residue.

The lesson of the drawings by Ukrainian students might be that, whether we wish it or not, the war will continue even during peacetime. As long as we remember, we are still in ruins. The images convey ideas in the form of fragments, as metonymical representations of a sense of loss that cannot be realised exhaustively. By pointing to this sense of loss in sketches, as if they opened the singularity of the lived experience, the depictions produce an invaluable archive of reactions to the war. The moments embraced by the images are at once immediate, exact and incidental. Their symbolic elements and cultural codes speak to viewers, but this speech is mute, unforeseeable and makes us responsible for what we perceive. The ruined sights lack words, and when we resort to words, they cannot be but our own, telling truths that are always only partial and fractured.[13]

Notes

1 In Greek, *helios* means 'sun' and *anthus* is the word for 'flower'. *Annuus* refers to the Latin word for 'year', as sunflower is an annual forb.
2 In Derrida's philosophy, the 'trait' denotes, in its most concrete sense, the outcome of a draughtsman's work: the line of a drawing. It may also signify feature, stroke, mark, tracing, outline and trace. Along with these meanings, the trait has another, more abstract sense: it is the possibility to leave traces. A similar ambiguity belongs to Derrida's concepts of 'writing' and 'arche-writing'. See Derrida, 1991/1993, pp. 2–3.
3 See also Owens, 1979, pp. 43–45.
4 Especially in a written work, the 'scattered fragments' are an alteration of the Latin phrase *disjecti membra poetae*. These words were used by Horace (65–8 BCE) in *Satires* (2012, 1.4.62): '[In our case] you would not [as you would in the case of those Ennian lines] find the limbs of a dismembered poet'.
5 Of the heart's familiarity and strangeness, see Nancy, 1992/2008, pp. 161–170.
6 From the Middle Ages to the Renaissance and onwards, from paintings by Hieronymus Bosch (*Visions of the Hereafter*, 1505–1515), Jan Brueghel the Elder, Giotto and Michelangelo (*The Torment of St Anthony*, 1487–1488) to Odilon Redon's fantastic species in the late nineteenth and early twentieth

century, devils are tempting Christ, saints or ordinary humans to evil or causing nightmares and disasters. See e.g. 'The devil you know in paintings'.

7 Behind Kant's notion of 'radical evil' is the Christian term *radix malorum* (Kant, 1793–1794/2009).

8 The saying appears already in Cicero (106–43 BCE) who is quoted as saying 'Ut imago est animi voltus sic indices oculi'—'The face is a picture of the mind as the eyes are its interpreter'.

9 According to Abraham Maslow's hierarchy of needs, food, water, clothing, sleep and shelter are the basic physiological necessities for living. Above them are the higher-level psychological needs, such as safety, belonging and love, esteem, cognitive and aesthetic needs, self-actualisation and, finally, transcendence (Maslow, 1943).

10 Atkinson notes that Derrida's idea of the inaccessible, ghost-like nature of trauma differs from the view of Nicolas Abraham and Mária Török, Hungarian-born French psychoanalysts who worked extensively on trauma from the 1950s to 1970s. According to Abraham and Török, like a phantom, trauma resides in a 'crypt', a gap of knowledge that is of subjective origin, whereas for Derrida there is never a common subjective 'crypt' for trauma, hence it is too singular and, at the same time, too placeless to be spoken out. Abraham and Török's attempt to make the unspeakable speak seems, for Derrida, a doubtful attempt (Derrida, 1977/1986, p. xvi).

11 About the theme of barbarism, see also Hullot-Kentor, 2010, pp. 23–42.

12 In Jean-François Lyotard's philosophy, the concept of differend signals an unsolvable event, a situation where the discordant parties cannot be returned to the sphere of the same (Lyotard, 1983/1988).

13 I thank Kone Foundation for the financial support of my research during 2021–2023.

References

Adorno, T. W. (1967). Cultural criticism and society (S. Weber & S. Weber, Trans.). In T. W. Adorno (Ed.), *Prisms: Essays in cultural criticism and society* (pp. 17–34). Spearman. (Original work published 1951)

Atkinson, M. (2013). Channeling the specter and translating phantoms: Hauntology and the spooked text. In M. Atkinson & M. Richardson (Eds.), *Traumatic affect* (pp. 247–270). Cambridge Scholars Publishing.

Bisson, J. I., Cosgrove, S., Lewis, C. & Robert, N. P. (2015). Post-traumatic stress disorder. *BMJ, 351*, h6161.

Derrida, J. (1986). Foreword: *Fors*: The Anglish words of Nicolas Abraham and Maria Torok. In N. Abraham & M. Török (Eds.), *The Wolf Man's magic word: A cryptonomy* (pp. xi–xlviii). University of Minnesota Press. (Original work published 1977)

Derrida, J. (1987). *The truth in painting* (G. Bennington & I. McLeod, Trans.). The University of Chicago Press. (Original work published 1978)

Derrida, J. (1993). *Memoirs of the blind: The self-portrait and other ruins* (P.-A. Brault & M. Naas, Trans.). The University of Chicago Press. (Original work published 1991)

Derrida, J. (1994). *The specters of Marx* (P. Kamuf, Trans.). Routledge. (Original work published 1993)

Derrida, J. (2010). *Athens, still remains* (P.-A. Brault & M. Naas, Trans.). Fordham University Press. (Original work published 1996)

Derrida, J. (2021). Drawing by design (L. Milesi, Trans.). In G. Michaud, J. Masó & J. Bassas (Eds.), *Thinking out of sight: Writings on the arts of the visible* (pp. 98–117). The University of Chicago Press. (Original work published 1991)

Foltynova, K. (2022, December 24). Protecting the skies: How does Ukraine defend against Russian missiles? *Radio Free Europe / Radio Liberty.* https://www.rferl.org/a/ukraine-missile-defense-weapons-charts-russia/32192132.html

Horace (2012). *Satires, Book I* (E. Gowers, Trans.). Cambridge University Press.

Hullot-Kentor, R. (2010) What barbarism is? In F. Akcelrud Durão (Ed.), *Culture industry today* (pp. 23–42). Cambridge Scholars Publishing.

Kant, I. (1993). *Groundwork of the metaphysics of morals* (J. W. Ellington, Trans.). Hackett. (Original work published 1785)

Kant, I. (2009). *Religion within the bounds of bare reason* (W. S. Pluhar, Trans.). Hackett. (Original work published 1793–1794)

Lyotard, J.-F. (1988). *The differend* (G. Van Den Abbeele, Trans.). University of Minnesota Press. (Original work published 1983)

Maslow, A. (1943). A theory of human motivation. *Psychological Review, 50*(4), 370–396.

Nancy, J.-L. (2008). *Corpus* (R. A. Rand, Trans.). Fordham University Press. (Original work published 1992)

Nosthoff, A.-V. (2014, October 15). Barbarism: Notes on the thought of Theodor W. Adorno. *Critical Legal Thinking.* https://criticallegalthinking.com/2014/10/15/barbarism-notes-thought-theodor-w-adorno/

Owens, C. (1979). Detachment from the *parergon. October, 9*(Summer), 42–49.

Plato (1997). Republic (G. M. A. Grube & C. D. C. Reeve, Trans.). In J. M. Cooper (Ed.), *Complete works* (pp. 971–1223). Hackett.

'The devil you know in paintings'. (2019, January 19). *The Eclectic Light Company.* https://eclecticlight.co/2019/01/19/the-devil-you-know-in-paintings-1/.

Wulfeck, A. (2022, March 10). Why the sunflower has grown in popularity during the Russia-Ukraine conflict. *The New York Post.* https://nypost.com/2022/03/10/why-the-sunflower-has-grown-in-popularity-during-the-russia-ukraine-conflict/

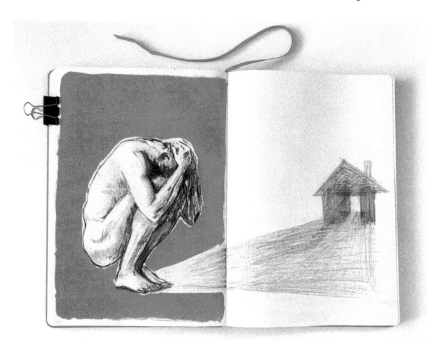

IMAGE 6.1   Eva Alvor. (2022). Eskiz2.

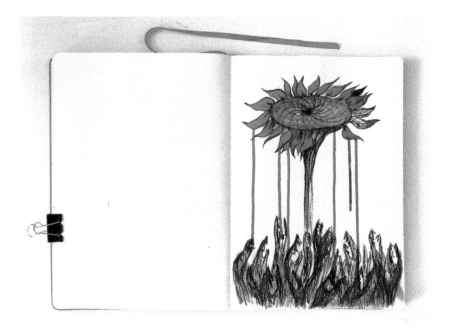

IMAGE 6.2   Eva Alvor. (2022). Eskiz6.

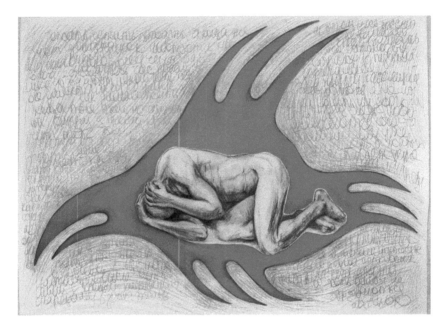

IMAGE 6.3 Eva Alvor. (2022). Tryvoga.

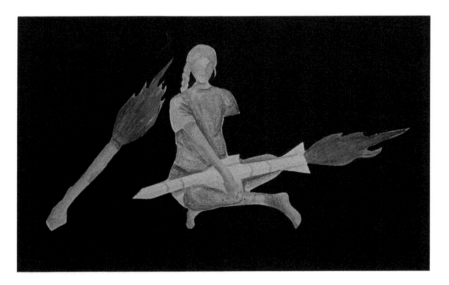

IMAGE 6.4 Anastasiia B. (2022). Untitled image.

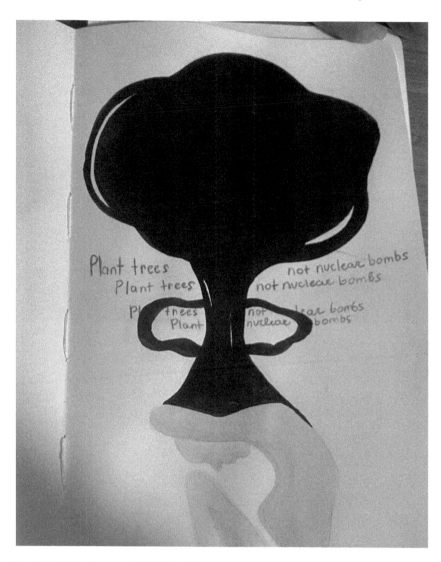

IMAGE 6.5   Anastasiia B. (2022). Untitled image.

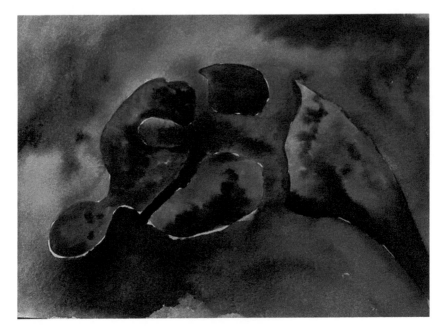

IMAGE 6.6 Anastasiia B. (2022). Untitled image.

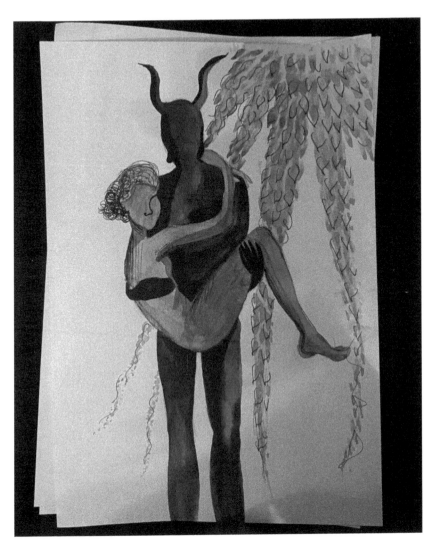

IMAGE 6.7 Anastasiia B. (2022). Untitled image.

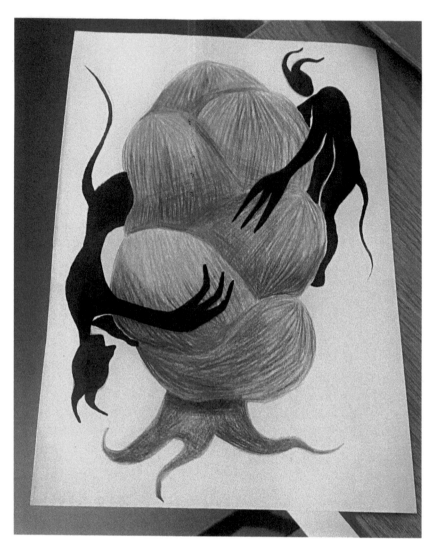

IMAGE 6.8 Anastasiia B. (2022). Untitled image.

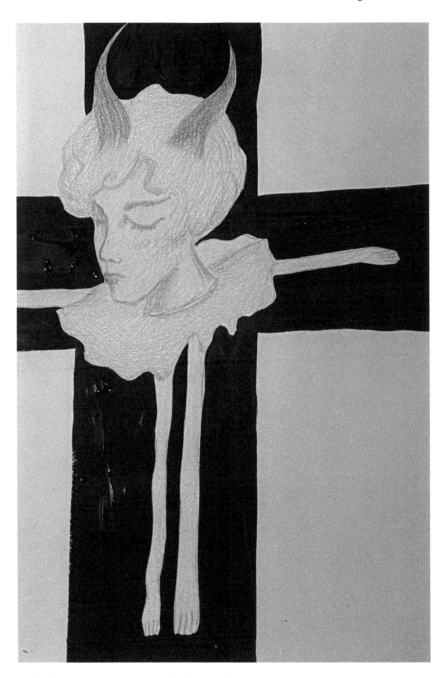

IMAGE 6.9 Anastasiia B. (2022). Untitled image.

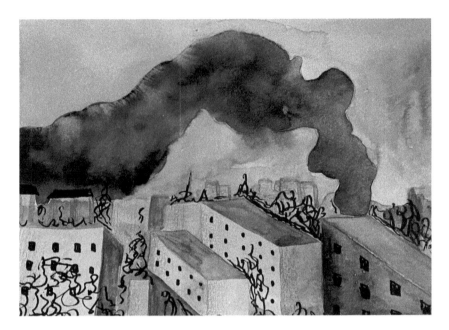

IMAGE 6.10 Anastasiia B. (2022). Untitled image.

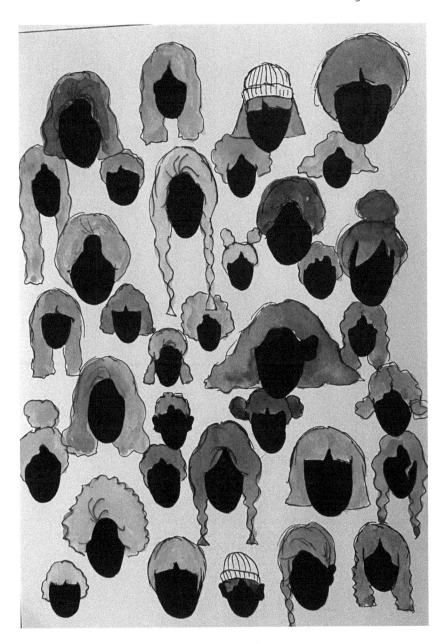

IMAGE 6.11 Anastasiia B. (2022). Untitled image.

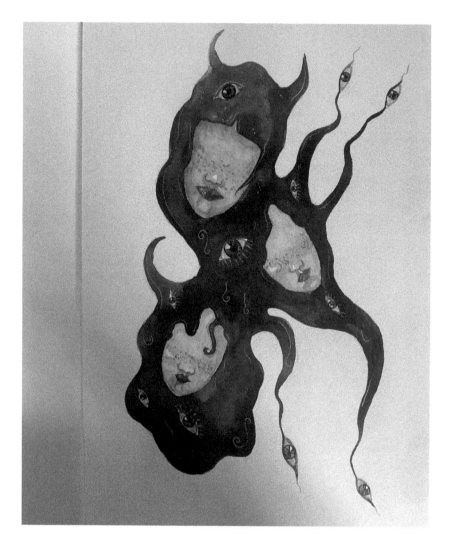

IMAGE 6.12 Anastasiia B. (2022). Untitled image.

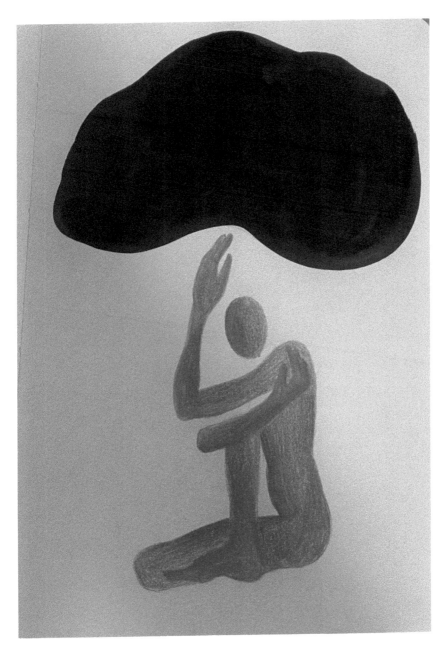

IMAGE 6.13 Anastasiia B. (2022). Untitled image.

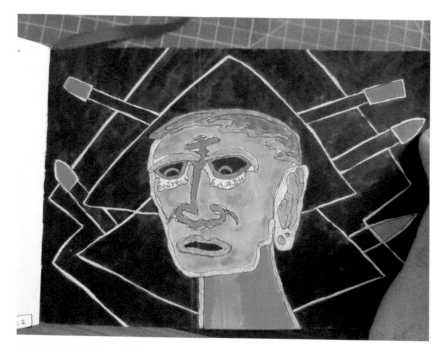

IMAGE 6.14 Ihor Kolesnyk. (2022). Untitled image.

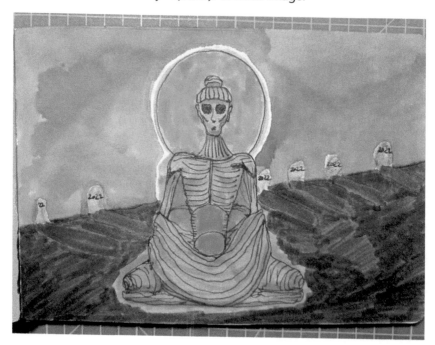

IMAGE 6.15 Ihor Kolesnyk. (2022). Untitled image.

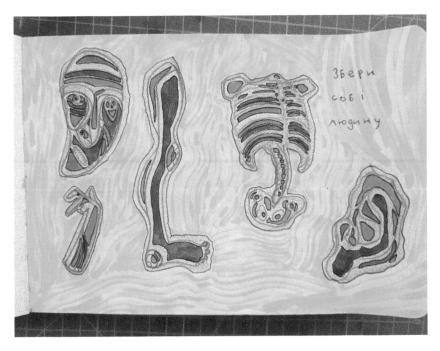

IMAGE 6.16   Ihor Kolesnyk. (2022). Untitled image.

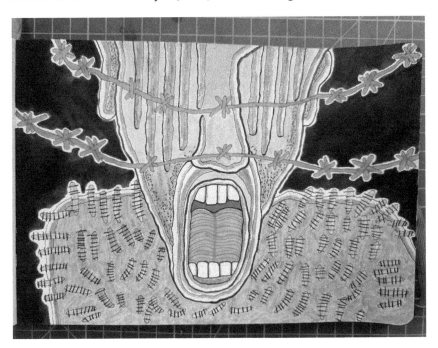

IMAGE 6.17   Ihor Kolesnyk. (2022). Untitled image.

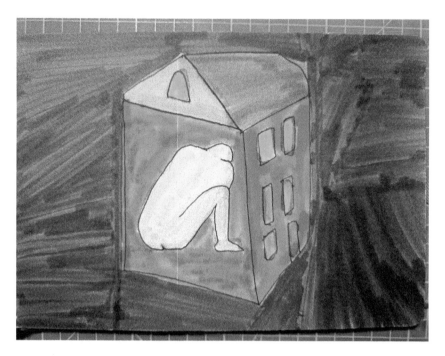

IMAGE 6.18 Ihor Kolesnyk. (2022). Untitled image.

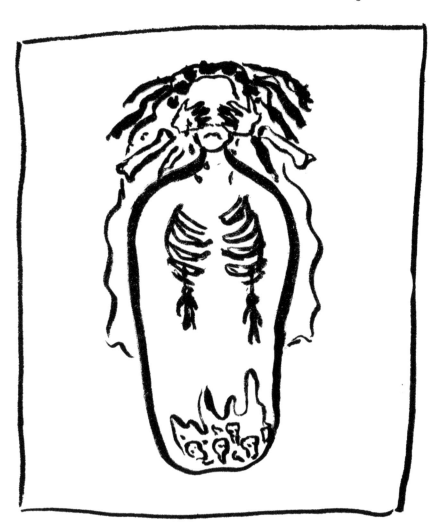

IMAGE 6.19 Kateryna Luzganova. (2022). Untitled image.

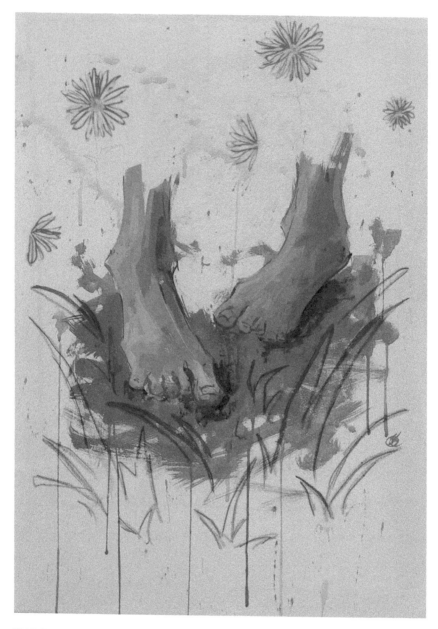

IMAGE 6.20 Uliana Pasternak (2022). Untitled image.

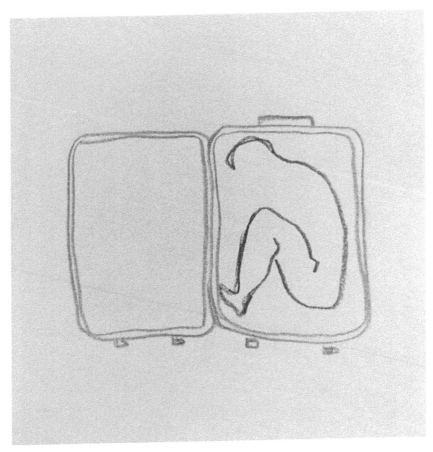

IMAGE 6.21 Uliana Pasternak. (2022). Untitled image.

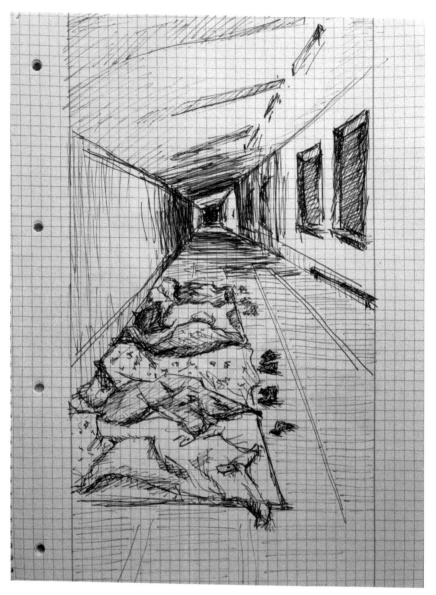

IMAGE 6.22 Marharita Zavhorodnia. (2022). Untitled image.

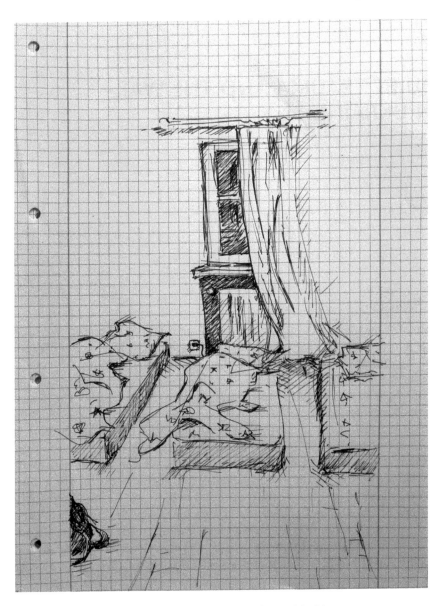

IMAGE 6.23   Marharita Zavhorodnia. (2022). Untitled image.

7

QUIET TRAUMA AND THE WAR IN UKRAINE

Chari Larsson

Introduction

One of the striking recurring themes characterising the *Diaries of War and Life* photography project is the participants' willingness to open their homes and apartments with the spectator. This is a gesture of generosity and a willingness to share. For example, there is something remarkably familiar about Stefaniia Kolesnyk's photograph (Image 7.1, p. 174). The image shows two women in an apartment. One is kneeling and the other is lying on her stomach on a couch with her head supported by her hand. There is something friendly and relaxed about the image, as if the women have invited us in to visit and are disclosing a private moment of their time. Both women are smiling for the camera, and it is not clear whether there is a third person, the photographer, or the camera has been set to an auto-timer. There is a pile of blankets and pillows on the sofa suggesting an impromptu 'sleep over'. To the left, there is an entranceway leading to the apartment's front door. The wall behind the couch is bare. The photograph's depth of field is shallow, and our eyes return to the women. This has an effect of reinforcing the intimacy of the photograph's composition. The image's informality is enhanced by its unarranged composition: the women have not taken the time to organise the bedding into a neat pile. Slowly, signs of defiance begin to emerge. The crouching woman holds her hand in the 'V' for Victory hand signal, however, it is unclear as to whether this is a friendly signal directed towards the spectator, or something more rebellious.

How do we begin to approach the impact of trauma on both individuals and entire nations? The *Diaries of War and Life* photography project developed by students and staff at the Lviv Centre for Urban History is a

DOI: 10.4324/9781003449096-11

visual chronicle of the confusion and turmoil of the earliest days of Russia's full-scale invasion in February 2022. Geographically distant from Ukraine's front lines in the East and South, Lviv has provided security and refuge for internally displaced Ukrainians, as well as a crucial departure hub for those seeking asylum. The collection sits somewhat awkwardly in relation to existing paradigms of war photography. Instead, the images are closer to what photographic historians have defined as 'vernacular' photography, or ordinary photographs taken by ordinary people. There is nothing ordinary, however, about war.

My chapter will proceed in two sections. In the first, I wish to draw together the notoriously slippery categories of vernacular photography and the everyday. Working in a vernacular mode of address, the photographic images in the *Diaries of War and Life* collection are akin to a visual diary: highly personal records of the strange otherworldliness accompanying the chaos and upheaval of the war in Ukraine. My chapter investigates the relationship between trauma, vernacular photography, and the documentation of the everyday and asks how this project might yield new forms of representing traumatic experience. I wish to interrogate the conditions of visibility of a contemporary archive, to understand how the collection challenges longer histories of the gaze and spectatorship that have been predicated on suspicion and hostility. My hypothesis here is the ubiquity of smartphone technology has facilitated a new, emerging mode of visualising civilian trauma. Civilians can now document and share their experiences, away from the direct armed conflict using smartphones. The concept of 'quiet' trauma helps encapsulate this broad notion of community-based trauma.

The second section will ask what pressure do the images in the *Diaries of War and Life* collection exert on available models of spectatorship? I wish to reorientate a model of spectatorship around the concept of the friend (*philos*) as discussed by Indo-European linguist Émile Benveniste. Benveniste draws from Homer to demonstrate the original usage of the term is very different to its contemporary use. Benveniste's retrieval of the term *philos* helps us move beyond traditional modes of spectatorship predicated on suspicion and criticism. Departing from the existing categories determining war photography, the images attend to signs of defiance, as well as initiating a relationship with the spectator understood as a 'stranger-guest' that is predicated on hospitality.

War, Trauma and Vernacular Photography

Since February 2022, photographs taken by professional photojournalists have permeated our daily mediascapes. Images documenting the Battle of Kharkiv, the Siege of Mariupol, and the massacres at Bucha have been viewed with a mixture of compassion and a sensation of utter helplessness. Professional photojournalists will capture what will, in time, be regarded as iconic war images (Hariman & Lucaites, 2007). These images will distil the essence of the invasion, its toll on the civilian population, and the catastrophic humanitarian disaster that has unfolded. An everyday account of war, however, sits apart from highly recognisable categories such as atrocity photographs, or the auteur trademark styles of well-known photojournalists representing international organisations such as Lynsey Addario or Emilio Morenatti. If photojournalists are charged with the responsibility of capturing iconic war images, how may we begin to approach images that do not conform to the conventions demanded by iconic or atrocity photography, but are taken by citizens who are obviously suffering from various degrees of trauma?

One of the most important aspects of trauma is defining it. Trauma theory in its psychoanalytic and poststructuralist forms has stressed the unrepresentable and inaccessible nature of traumatic experience. Emerging in the context of Holocaust research, this line of thought emerged in the 1990s and became primarily associated with literary theorists such as Cathy Caruth. For Caruth, trauma is 'unassimilable to consciousness' (1996, p. 116). Any attempt to represent trauma will inevitably fail, as the traumatic event can only be understood belatedly. Another important point of reference is Dori Laub and Shoshana Felman's *Testimony: Crises of Witnessing in Literature, Psychoanalysis, and History* (1992). Laub and Felman also describe something that is 'beyond' representation, or the 'shock of the unintelligible in the face of the attempt at its interpretation' (1992, p. xx).

Whilst trauma's moment of 'high' theory might have passed, there is little doubt that the need to continue theorising the nature of traumatic experience has not. If the traumatic experience yields a breakdown in representation, what role might photography play? If the first generation of theorists emphasised trauma's inability to be represented, the *Diaries of War and Life* project is moving in precisely the opposite direction. Smartphones facilitate a diaristic visual account of the participants' experiences and observations. The images are diverse in their subject matter and oscillate between exercising a pet to subjects more aligned with traditional war photography such as sheltering underground, or taping windows to try and protect an apartment's windows from shattering in a drone or missile attack. In his preface to *The Future of Trauma Theory*, Michael Rothberg has argued that the '"new" trauma theory' is still in the process of developing new theoretical paradigms to build on its classical predecessors (2014, p. xii). What is needed is a new vocabulary for considering the lived experience of civilians in war. Responding to Rothberg's provocation, I argue that the *Diaries of War and Life* project is a visual chronicle of civilian trauma, or what I will call 'quiet' trauma. The collection is highly personal and works in an affectual register akin to its literary equivalent, the diary.

The concept of 'quiet trauma' was discussed by Ann E. Kaplan in *Trauma Culture* (2005). In the text she observes that stress is not just limited to soldiers fighting on the front lines, but also impacts relatives on the home front (p. 1). I wish to expand the concept beyond immediate relatives to include communities that have been impacted by the terror of war, but not necessarily living in the combat zones. Quiet trauma is given visual form in the *Diaries of War and Life* collection via a variety of aesthetic strategies. Frequently, at first glance, everything appears 'normal'. On closer inspection, however, it appears that routine life has been bracketed or deferred. Ruta Randmaa, for instance, chronicled the preventative measures taken to safeguard historical and cultural monuments in Lviv's Old Town (Image 7.2, p. 175). Statues have been wrapped and are encased by scaffolding to minimise damage in an attack. In other images, church stained-glass windows have been boarded up with plywood (Image 7.3, p. 176). There is an elegiac, mournful tone associated with this series of photographs, and it is this suspension of everyday life and the associated community response where we must begin to locate the project.

The methods and technologies used to visually document the war in Ukraine have changed since earlier wars. Smartphone technology was still in its embryonic forms during the wars in Iraq. Commencing in 2014 with the annexation of Crimea and the Russian-backed conflict in the Donbas region, the war in Ukraine is the first conflict where smartphone use is nearly ubiquitous amongst the civilian population. Civilians can now document and share their everyday experiences, away from the frontlines. Consider, for example, Anastasiia Markeliuk's sequence. Located in a darkened interior, Markeliuk's photographs move closer to art photography rather than the traditional documentary style adopted by the other participants (Images 7.4–7.5, p. 177–178). In this series, Anastasiia Markeliuk has overlaid images onto larger images, creating internal dialogues. Close-ups of feet and toes are juxtaposed with a figure sitting on a chair, reading a smartphone (Image 7.6, p. 179).

The visualisation of civilian or 'quiet' trauma is distinctly at odds with the history of war photography that privileges highly recognisable genres. Marta Zarzycka (2016) has argued that tropes such as the mourning woman, the wounded soldier, and refugee mother and child have recurred across historical periods and function as generic media templates. Amateur photojournalism and the use of smartphones have allowed for the documentation of the invasion in cities such as Bucha where international media could not enter (Stallabrass, 2022, p. 8). The *Diaries of War and Life* project is unusual because it bears little resemblance to both of these categories.

The collection is comprised of what we *don't* see in the media. The images are not determined by violence, death, or atrocity. Instead, the participants tend to be working in a highly personal manner, eschewing documentary photography's preference for objectivity.

In this way, the images are akin to highly personal visual diaries. Diaries are usually private, a record of our most intimate thoughts. Visual diaries are no different. The decision to share with the spectator is an incredibly generous action, as diaries enjoy a privileged rapport with the 'truth'. Philippe Lejeune (2009) coined the neologism 'antifiction' to describe this relationship:

> Diarists never have control over what comes next in their texts. They write with no way of knowing what will happen next in the plot, much less how it will end. The past is wonderfully malleable [...]. The future is pitiless and the unforeseeable. And the present—the diarist's subject matter—immediately objects to anything that smacks of invention. (p. 202)

Diary writing is considered by Lejeune as preferable to autobiography, because of its commitment to truth-telling. Writing in the present demands an accuracy or truth-telling that is not shared by its adjacent literary genres, autobiography and memoire. As Lejeune playfully puts it: 'The diary grows weak and faints or breaks out in a rash when it comes into contact with fiction' (2009, p. 204).

The photographs in the *Diaries of War and Life* collection belong to a genre that photographic historians termed 'vernacular photography', or photographs taken by ordinary people often of everyday things. Vernacular photography has sat awkwardly outside of 'official' photographic histories. As Geoffrey Batchen observed, 'vernaculars are photography's *parergon*, the part of its history that has been pushed to the margins (2000, p. 262). Clément Chéroux also notes that vernacular photography 'flourishes at the margins' (2020, p. 25). The everyday, as an academic category, is another notoriously slippery category. In his first volume of the *Critique of Everyday Life*, Henri Lefebvre famously defined everyday life as 'in a sense residual, defined by "what is left over" after all distinct, superior, specialized, structured activities that have been singled out by analysis' (1947/1991, p. 97). The *Diaries of War and Life* collection might be best understood as 'what is left over' from the categories of war images produced for the mainstream media. In this context, the everyday is understood positively, as an embrace of the mundane and overlooked. Civilian documentation of the everyday during war tends to typically be comprised of the unnoticed, trivial and prosaic or repetitive aspects of daily life.

One of the most ubiquitous forms of everyday portraiture to emerge with the use of smartphones is the selfie. In Ihor Kolesnyk's self-portrait (Image 7.7, p. 180), we are presented with another casual snapshot. Ihor has taken a selfie with his cat who is nestled inside his sweater and lazily peers in the direction of the camera. Given the arm's length distance of the selfie, we are presented with a close-up of his face, which dominates the camera's frame. The image has been taken in an interior as we are given a glimpse of the earthy tones and vertical stripes of a sofa and the verticality of a wall that forecloses any sense of deep space. Ihor Kolesnyk does not quite make direct eye contact with the viewer. Instead, his eyes are slightly directed towards the bottom left corner of the image. Intimacy is enhanced by the spectator's close physical proximity to Ihor, and we are left to study his facial structure without directly encountering his gaze. The cat appears hairless, creating an unexpected juxtaposition with Ihor's beard and hair, which dominate the image. In this case, the selfie is behaving much like a highly personal diary entry, capturing a specific moment in time.

I was struck by the signals of national pride and resistance that are woven through the collection. Sometimes, these are ambiguous. For instance, in Stefaniia Kolsenyk's photograph (Image 7.1, p. 174), the interior palette is punctuated with yellows and blues, the colours of the Ukrainian flag. The bed cover is yellow and is juxtaposed with the blues of the women's jeans, tracksuit pants and sofa. It is uncertain as to whether this is a 'happy accident', or something more deliberate. Alternatively, consider Yevheniia Marchuk's remarkable self-portrait taken whilst walking her dog in the countryside (Image 7.8, p. 181). Like the other photographs in the collection, the image is disarming because of its everyday familiarity as we can connect with our own experiences or memories of exercising pets. Marchuk registers her physical presence in the photograph through her shadow, which looms slightly to the centre-left. The viewer's eye is directed immediately down the road which is framed by the remnants of a crop. Strikingly, the composition of the photograph is evocative of the Ukrainian flag. The strong horizontal line divides the image between the blue of the sky and the yellow, brownish tones of the field below. Signs of Ukrainian resistance are imprinted on the landscape itself.

Other examples of Ukrainian pride are not quite as oblique. Ruta Randmaa photographed a signed Ukrainian flag (Image 7.9, p. 182). Presumably, the signatures belong to soldiers who have been deployed to combat on the front line. Bohdana Serdiukova's images (Images 7.10–7.11, pp. 183–184) document anti-Russian protests and rallies she attended and spoke at whilst living in Sweden. In one image, she wears a blue and yellow ribbon tied around her neck (Image 7.12, p. 184). In other photographs, resistance and resilience are demonstrated through her use of fashion

(Image 7.13, p. 185). In several images, she and others wear shirts and dresses adorned with the vyshyvanka, a traditional type of Ukrainian embroidery (Serdiukova, Image 7.14, p. 186; Clarin, Image 7.15, p. 187). Fashion is used here pointedly in protest as Ukrainians were outlawed by the Soviet regime for wearing vyshyvanka in the 1950s and 1960s (Wong, 2023).

Lurking around the edges of the collection is the threat of violence. Olena Pohonchenkova has captured the visible alterations and changes made to her apartment in case of a missile or drone attack (Image 7.16, p. 188). The windows have been covered with blankets to help protect from shards of glass becoming potential weapons. In other photographs, Pohonchenkova concentrates on recording the experience of those seeking refuge in the underground hallways at the Lviv railway station and emergency shelters that have been set up throughout the city (Images 7.17–7.18, p. 189–190). Railway stations were famously declared 'non-places' by Marc Augé (1992/1995). Olena Pohonchenkova's sequence transforms this description, and the railway station is instead visualised as a place providing shelter and security.

There is a documentary impulse at work in this series, and many of her photographs have focused on the details of personal objects people have carried with them. For example, in one photograph, there appears to be an enormous sieve and it is balanced on large containers that might have once held flour (Image 7.19, p. 191). The photograph has been cropped so that we cannot see the subject's head. Instead, we are left with a glimpse of a book that they are reading whilst sheltering. The shift of emphasis from subject to object has the effect of subtly differentiating the sequence from the flood of media images that tend to be easily 'read'. Instead, the spectator's gaze is frustrated: the technique encourages a fragmentary, distorted effect as the images refuse to adhere to a coherent narrative. Other images in Olena Pohonchenkova's collection focus on rows of blankets that have been set down on the hard cold floor of the train station and we are reminded of the role Lviv has played as a humanitarian hub since the earliest days of the invasion (Image 7.20, p. 192).

In her collection of photographs, Olena Pohonchenkova has included a self-portrait. Instead of a narcissistic or exhibitionist performance of the self, Olena's selfie in this context is something closer to evidence: 'I was here, seeking shelter. This is proof' (Image 7.21, p. 193). In this way, Olena's self-portrait is redolent of Roland Barthes' observations pertaining to photography's referentiality. In *Camera Lucida*, Barthes referred to this idea as the 'That-has-been' or photography's *noeme* (1980/1984, p. 77). It is the photograph's proof that someone existed. I am deliberately returning here to an older, pre-digital account of photography where the referent still 'adheres' (Barthes, 1980/1984, p. 6). I would like to underscore the selfie's capacity to bear witness, to document the everyday made strange through war.

The Spectator as 'Guest-Stranger'

What duty of care does the spectator owe a photographic 'archive' of the present tense? Unlike historical archives that provide a temporal distance between the researcher and the material, this archival collection exists in the present and is chronicling an event that is unfolding in real time. What modes of spectatorship are available to us? The traditional model of photojournalism was predicated on the photographer in the privileged position as 'witness' whose task was to educate and inform the viewer. When we shift our attention to vernacular images, ethical questions are immediately raised pertaining to what it means to take photographs at sites of trauma. Writing in the direct aftermath of 9/11, Marianne Hirsch asks, 'But what does it mean to take pictures at the sites of trauma? Is it disrespectful, voyeuristic, a form of gawking? Or is it our own contemporary form of witnessing or even mourning?' (2003, p. 71). In a similar vein, Ann E. Kaplan described her propulsion to photograph and document:

> In the shocked days after the Twin Towers collapsed and thousands of people died in unimaginable ways, I wandered around my neighbourhood between Union Square and SoHo, trying to absorb what had happened. My camera was my only companion. I snapped pictures (sometimes feeling guilty—was I invading people's privacy?) in an attempt, I think, to make "real" what I could barely comprehend. (2005, p. 2)

Both anecdotes suggest that one possible coping mechanism for victims of quiet trauma is to document via photography.

If we turn to photographic discourse itself, the nexus between trauma, photography, and spectatorship is deeply ambivalent. Decades ago, Susan Sontag famously mused, 'Images transfix. Images anesthetize' (1973, p. 20). What does it mean to look repeatedly at images taken by civilians who are quietly suffering and at what point does the compassion fatigue described by Sontag inevitably impact our ability to look? Sontag took up the question again, this time problematising the role of the photographer. For Sontag, the camera may 'presume, intrude, trespass, distort, exploit' (1973, p. 13). Susie Linfield has argued that photography's history is characterised by a deep suspicion. Linfield develops a genealogical history that spans twentieth-century theorists such as Sontag and Roland Barthes through to post-modernist and feminist accounts by photographers Allan Sekula and Martha Rosler. This leads Linfield to conclude that photography's most influential observers 'don't really like photographs, or the act of looking at them, at all' (2010, p. 5). Working in contradiction to this, the photographs in the *Diaries of War and Life* collection elude charges of suspicion or distrust, *because* of their familiarity and their preparedness to share with the spectator.

An example of this is Bohdana Serdiukova's series, which takes the form of a diarised account of her experience of the invasion over the duration of three months. Bohdana Serdiukova elected to combine text with images. This creates a linear narrative structure, as well as providing context to her photographs. The first image in the sequence is taken at an airport. She is visiting her boyfriend who lives in Sweden. Surrounded by two bags, the photograph registers as normal, commemorating a moment of reunion (Image 7.22, p. 194). The next image is dated February 23 and Bohdana is standing in front of a low-rise apartment block and is being interviewed by a Swedish Radio station (Image 7.23, p. 194). On February 24, the date of the full-scale invasion: the following image is of Bohdana meeting online with Ukrainian children. 'I held a lesson with the children to calm them down' (Image 7.24, p. 195).

The visual and textual tone changes abruptly with the next image: 'Around 10:30 my mom called and said my dad was gone. I cried all day. I fell to the floor in horror' (Image 7.25, p. 195). Accompanying the text is a family photograph of Bohdana standing before the camera with her father. They both look directly at the camera. He has one arm wrapped around his daughter. She has her hand affectionately laid on his chest. The atmosphere shifts perceptibly to anguish as Bohdana attempts to make sense of her grief and physical distance to Ukraine and her mother. The sequence of images comprises of historical family portraits, selfies as well as photographs taken at demonstrations and rallies. Over the course of Bohdana Serdiukova's series, day-to-day activities gradually resume. The Swedish radio comes and interviews the children on their Zoom call. She documents the coming of Spring and the flowering of the cherry blossoms. According to the text entry accompanying the photograph, Bohdana is recreating a photograph of herself as a child.

One strategy that was developed specifically to engage with physical sites of trauma has been described as 'late' photography, or 'aftermath' photography (Baer, 2002; Campany, 2003/2007). French photographer Sophie Ristelhueber became emblematic of this aesthetic approach and tended to focus on the remnants or traces of an event that had taken place previously. This generally allows the photographer to circumvent accusations of fetishisation of human suffering and overidentification with the subject as a victim. In his analysis of the trend towards photographing the aftermath of events such as empty buildings and streets, David Campany has argued that this approach is closer to an aesthetic of 'forensic photography', rather than conventional photojournalism (2003/2007, p. 186). Working in a vernacular, diaristic manner is distinctly at odds with the deadpan, forensic aesthetic characterising aftermath photography. A vernacular mode of address actively solicits identification and empathy with the subject. Theorists of vernacular photography have sought to realign the relationship with the spectator with energetic and participatory forms of spectatorship. For instance, Batchen argued vernacular photography 'assumes the active involvement of the viewer as an interpretative agent' (2000, p. 268). Less preoccupied with a documentary 'truth' value assigned to documentary images, vernacular photographs instead perform social and cultural practices through their 'object-audience interaction' (Batchen, 2000, p. 268).

If we consider vernacular photography's calls for active spectatorship, the use of the smartphone invites a new line of enquiry. Writing specifically on the subject of amateurs' use of smartphones, Fred Ritchen has argued that smartphones offer a greater opportunity to create empathy with the spectator. He observes:

> These images constitute, to a certain extent, a common, diaristic dialect based on showing and sharing with cellphones—a language that is more detail-oriented and everyday, with fewer elaborately constructed attempts at the larger, synthesizing statement. (Ritchin, 2013, p. 11)

Extending Ritchen's observations, much of the *Diaries of War and Life* visual aesthetic is based on familiarity and intimacy. As viewers, we are invited into private domestic spaces and intimate moments that suggest an alternative model of viewing that is based on friendship and hospitality.

To develop this argument, I would like to retrieve Indo-European linguist Émile Benveniste's (1969/2016) study of the etymological history of friendship (*philos*). If we pursue Benveniste's etymological account of the term, it opens up an archaic understanding of friendship that is based on strict rules and conventions. Benveniste draws multiple examples from Homer to demonstrate how *philos* bears little resemblance to contemporary understandings of friendship with its association with sentimentality and affect. Alternatively, Benveniste argues that the Greek adjective *philos* is 'deeply rooted in the most ancient institutions of society and denotes a specific type of human relationship' (1969/2016, p. 283). For instance, in *The Odyssey*, Hermes has been sent by Zeus to the nymph Calypso and request Odysseus's release from her island. Calypso indignantly responds: 'But it was I who saved him [...] I fed him, loved him, sang that he should not die nor grow old, ever, in all the days to come' (1963, p. 5, 99). Calypso's point to Hermes is that as the host of her island, she was duty-bound to care for Odysseus after she rescued him drifting alone next to his ruined ship (1963, pp. 5, 94–96).

Benveniste elucidates an understanding of friendship that is closer to hospitality (*xénia*) and is best understood in terms of the rules or conventions that determine the behaviour towards a *xénos*, or guest. The verb *phileîn* (to be hospitable) is important as it is an expression of the rules or 'prescribed conduct' (1969/2016, p. 278) of the person who welcomes the *xénos* to his home. The relationship between host and guest is reciprocal. For instance,

Odysseus, now freed from Calypso's island, makes his way to Phaeacia. Here, he is a guest at Laodamas's house and is invited to demonstrate his sporting talents. Odysseus accepts the challenge, apart from Laodamas, whom he refuses to compete with:

> Racing, wrestling, boxing—I bar nothing with any man except Laodamas, for he's my host. Who quarrels with his host? Only a madman—or no man at all—would challenge his protector among strangers, cutting the ground away under his feet. (1963, p. 8, 173)

Philos, or friend, is understood as binding behaviour extended towards a *xénos*, or 'guest-stranger'. This relationship, argues Benveniste, is critical in the Homeric organisation of society (1969/2016, p. 278). Benveniste describes the relationship between host and guest as a 'pact' (1969/2016, p. 278). Crucially, as we have seen with the example of Odysseus and Laodamas, the pact is a two-way exchange.

This relationship allows us to begin sidestepping historical accounts of spectatorship that have been characterised by suspicion and distrust. Alternatively, it is the host's hospitality that welcomes us to view the photographic archive. As a guest, it is our duty and responsibility to reciprocate according to the Homeric conventions governing the relationship between host (*philos*) and guest (*xénos*). Benveniste emphasises the point: 'the notion of *philos* expresses the behavior incumbent on a member of the community towards a *xénos*, the "guest-stranger"' (1969/2016, p. 278). The connection between host and guest-stranger, or photographer and viewer, is governed by ancient rules or conventions. Following the logic of Benveniste's 'pact' helps structure our relationship with the *Diaries of War and Life* participants. This is a formal relationship that demands a distinct type of spectatorship: one that eschews both a scopophilic pleasure of looking, and alternatively a deep suspicion edging towards iconophobia.

In conclusion, the images in the *Diaries of War and Life* collection do not sit easily in existing paradigms of war photography. Instead, they are closely aligned to what has been defined as vernacular photography, or photographs taken by everyday people. In this chapter, I have argued that far from being unrepresentable, the process of creating, participating, and recording immediate responses to the Russian-Ukraine war demonstrates a departure from existing modes of spectatorship and witnessing, as well as the category of trauma itself. The images in the *Diaries of War and Life* project are an extraordinary act of generosity. It is our responsibility as a stranger-guest to return the gesture in the only way we have available to us: by looking and imagining. This is the duty of care that we, as guests, must bring when working with victims of quiet trauma.

References

Augé, M. (1995). *Non-places: Introduction to an anthropology of supermodernity* (J. Howe, Trans.). Verso. (Original work published 1992)

Baer, U. (2002). *Spectral evidence: The photography of trauma.* MIT Press.

Barthes, R. (1984). *Camera Lucida* (R. Howard, Trans.). Flamingo. (Original work published 1981)

Batchen, G. (2000). Vernacular photographies. *History of Photography, 24*(3), 262–271.

Benveniste, É. (2016). *Dictionary of Indo-European language and society* (E. Palmer, Trans.). Hau Books. (Original work published 1969)

Campany, D. (2003/2007). Safety in numbness: Some remarks on problems of 'late photography' (2003). In *The cinematic.* Whitechapel.

Caruth, C. (1996). *Unclaimed experience: Trauma, narrative, and history.* Johns Hopkins University Press.

Chéroux, C. (2020). Introducing Werner Kühler. In T. M. Campt, M. Hirsch, G. Hochberg & B. Wallis (Eds.), *Imagining everyday life: Engagements with vernacular photography* (pp. 22–31). Steidl, The Walther Collection.

Hariman, R. & Lucaites, J. L. (2007). *No caption needed: Iconic photographs, public culture, and liberal democracy.* University of Chicago Press.

Hirsch, M. (2003). I took pictures: September 2001 and beyond. In J. Greenberg (Ed.), *Trauma at home: After 9/11.* University of Nebraska Press.

Homer. (1963). *The odyssey* (R. Fitzgerald, Trans.). Anchor Books.

Kaplan, A. E. (2005). *Trauma culture: The politics of terror and loss in media and literature.* Rutgers University Press.

Laub, F. S. A. D. (1992). *Testimony: Crises of witnessing in literature, psychoanalysis, and history.* Routledge.

Lefebvre, H. (1991). *Critique of everyday life. Vol. 1: Introduction* (J. Moore, Trans.). Verso. (Original work published 1947)

Lejeune, P. (2009). The diary as "antifiction". In J. D. Popkin & J. Rak (Eds.), *On diary* (pp. 201–210). University of Hawaii Press.

Linfield, S. (2010). *The cruel radiance: Photography and political violence.* University of Chicago Press.

Ritchin, F. (2013). *Bending the frame: Photojournalism, documentary, and the citizen.* Aperture.

Rothberg, M. (2014). Preface: Beyond Tancred and Clorinda—trauma studies for implicated subjects. In G. Buelens, S. Durrant & R. Eaglestone (Eds.), *The future of trauma theory: Contemporary literary and cultural criticism* (pp. xi–xvii). Routledge.

Sontag, S. (1973). *On photography.* Farrar, Straus and Giroux.

Stallabrass, J. (2022). The look of war. *Art Monthly, 456,* 6–9.

Wong, F. (2023). *Fashion as protest in wartime: Ukrainian art as protest and resilience.* https://nanovic.nd.edu/features/fashion-as-protest-in-wartime/

Zarzycka, M. (2016). *Gendered tropes in war photography: Mothers, mourners, soldiers.* Routledge.

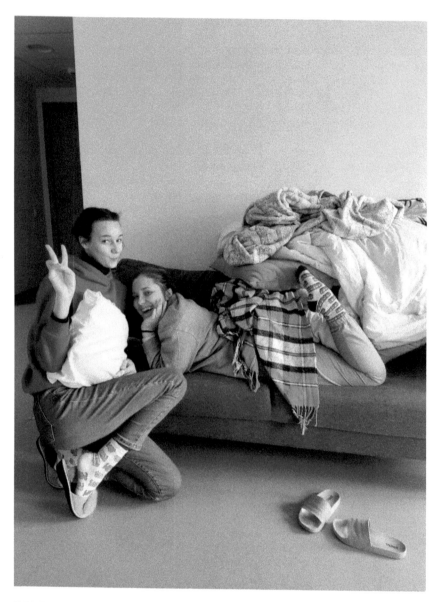

IMAGE 7.1 Stefaniia Kolesnyk. (March 07, 2022).

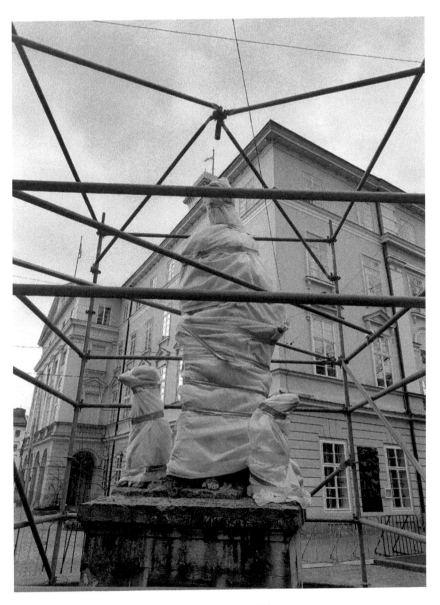

IMAGE 7.2 Ruta Randmaa. (March 10, 2022).

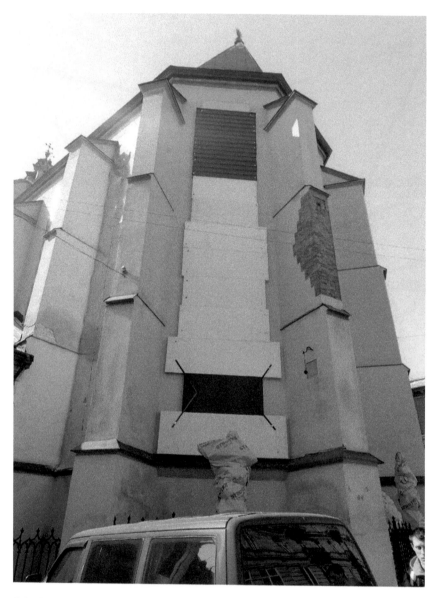

IMAGE 7.3 Ruta Randmaa. (April 16, 2022).

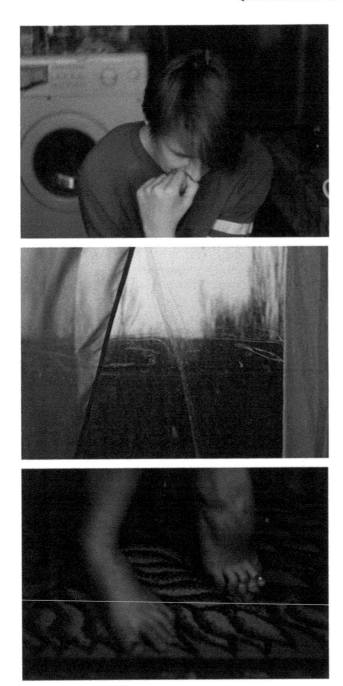

IMAGE 7.4 Anastasiia Markeliuk. (April 10, 2022).

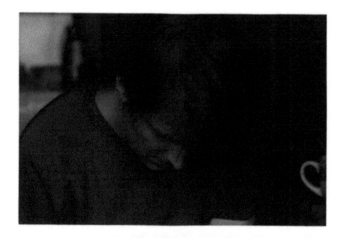

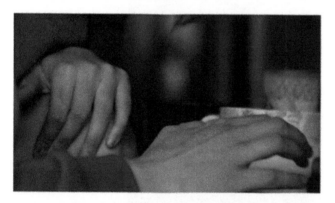

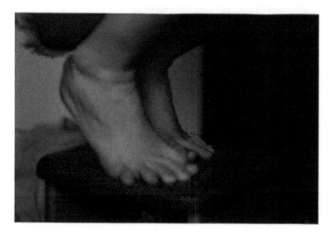

IMAGE 7.5 Anastasiia Markeliuk. (April 10, 2022).

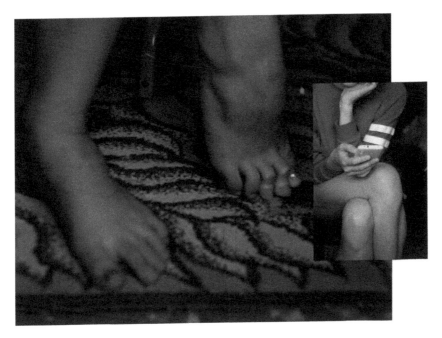

IMAGE 7.6   Anastasiia Markeliuk. (April 10, 2022).

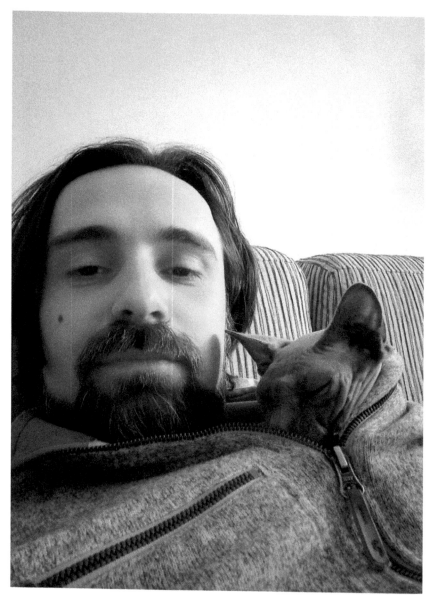

IMAGE 7.7 Ihor Kolesnyk. (March 15, 2022).

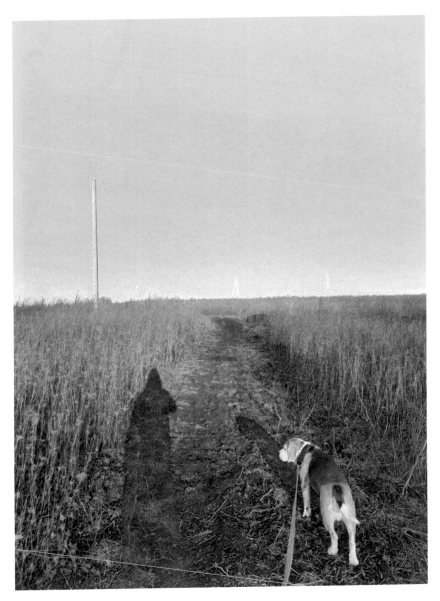

IMAGE 7.8 Yevheniia Marchuk. (2022).

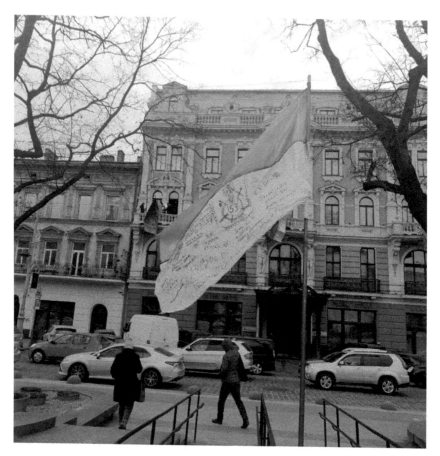

IMAGE 7.9 Ruta Randmaa. (March 10, 2022).

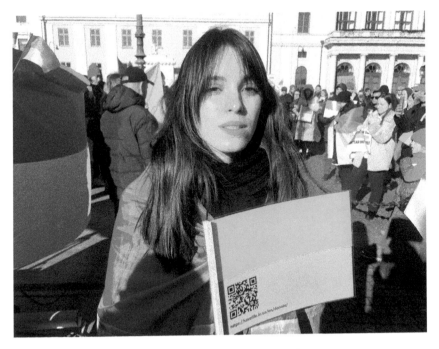

IMAGE 7.10 Bohdana Serdiukova. (May 13, 2022).

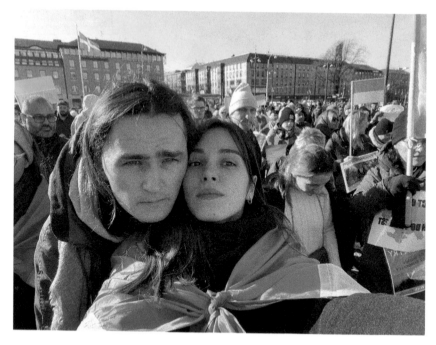

IMAGE 7.11   Bohdana Serdiukova. (May 13, 2022).

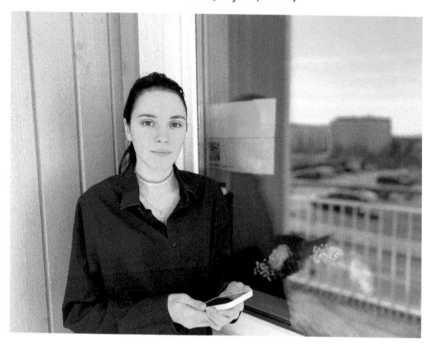

IMAGE 7.12   Bohdana Serdiukova. (May 13, 2022).

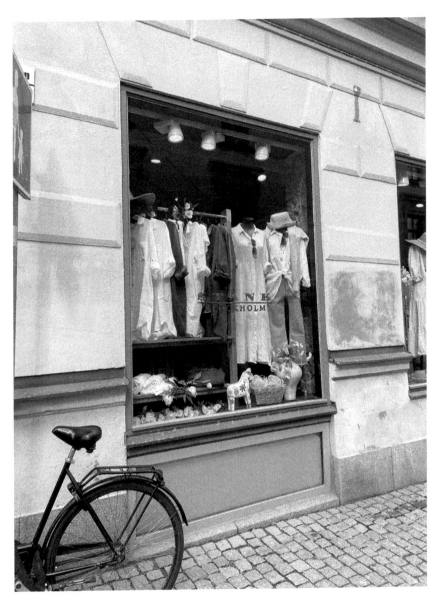

IMAGE 7.13   Bohdana Serdiukova. (May 13, 2022).

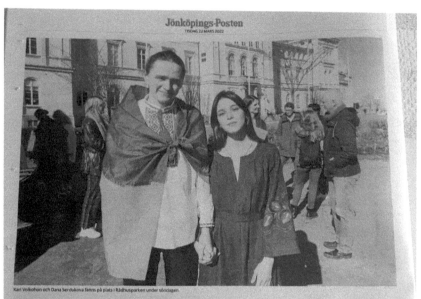

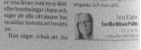

IMAGE 7.14   Bohdana Serdiukova. (May 13, 2022).

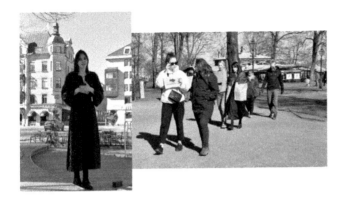

IMAGE 7.15   Lena Clarin. (May 13, 2022).

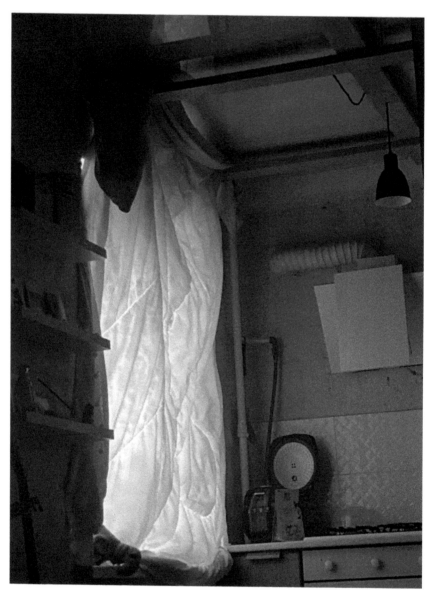

IMAGE 7.16 Olena Pohonchenkova. (March 10, 2022).

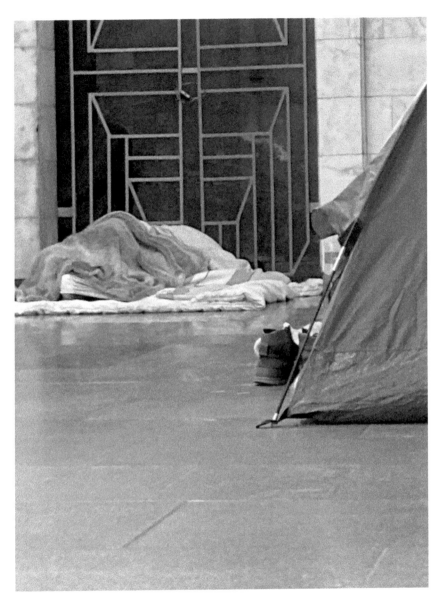

IMAGE 7.17 Olena Pohonchenkova. (March 10, 2022).

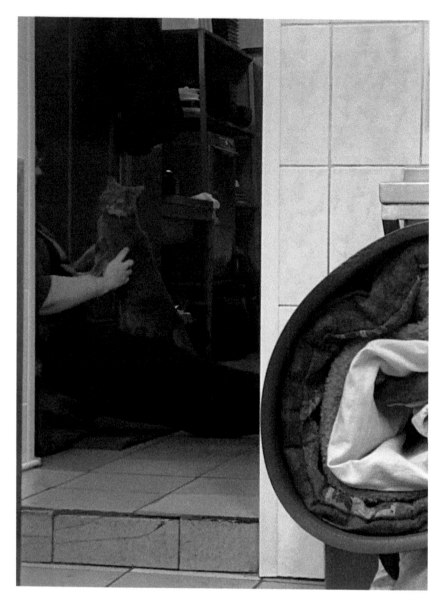

IMAGE 7.18 Olena Pohonchenkova. (March 10, 2022).

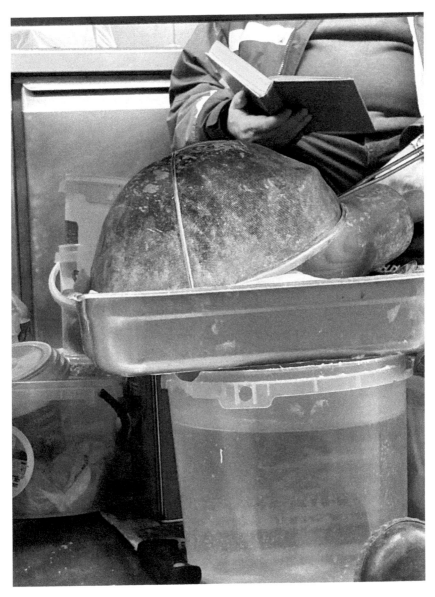

IMAGE 7.19 Olena Pohonchenkova. (March 10, 2022).

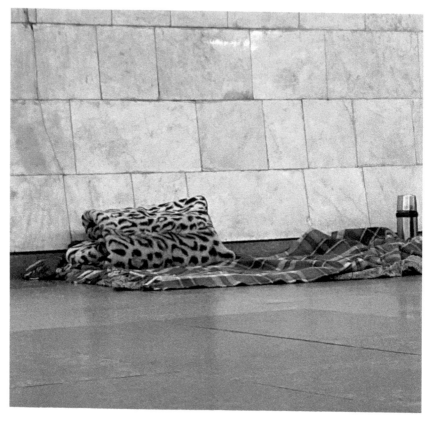

IMAGE 7.20 Olena Pohonchenkova. (March 10, 2022).

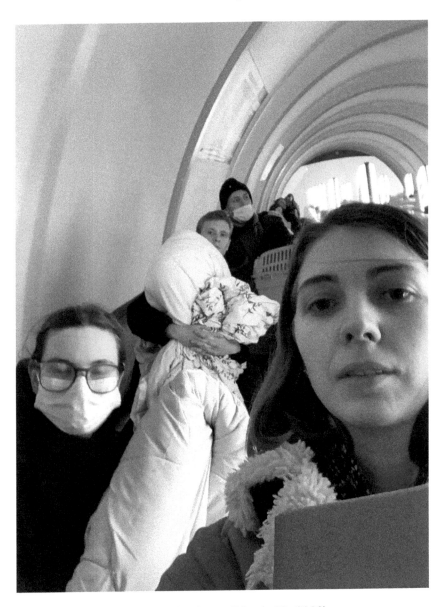

IMAGE 7.21 Olena Pohonchenkova. (March 10, 2022).

February 20.
I came to visit my boyfriend in Sweden

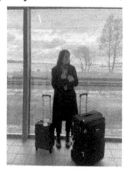

IMAGE 7.22   Bohdana Serdiukova. (February 20, 2022).

February 23
My boyfriend and I gave an
interview to Swedish radio

There was a lot of tension in the
news that day. So we were
asked: What do you think could
be the worst case scenario?
We said that the worst thing we
could imagine would be if our
parents were forced to leave
their homes and move
somewhere.

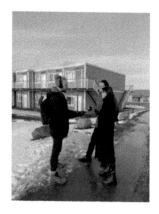

IMAGE 7.23   Bohdana Serdiukova. (February 23, 2022).

February 24, 9 a.m.
I held an online meeting with all the school children

I work as a school teacher and psychologist. At that meeting, I answered the children's questions and tried to give them as much support as possible.

At that time I did not know what had happened.

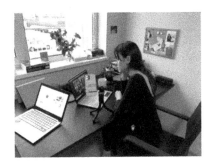

IMAGE 7.24   Bohdana Serdiukova. (February 24, 2022).

February 24. Around 10:30.
I got a call from my mother.
She said that my father had died.

I remember the feeling of horror, a lot of crying and screaming and that I was falling to the floor.
So much happened so quickly that I just couldn't take it.

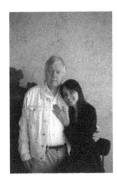

IMAGE 7.25   Bohdana Serdiukova. (February 24, 2022).

EXCERPTS FROM *DIARIES OF WAR AND LIFE (2)*

Anastasiia B.
February 24
Around 7 a.m.

I was eating pizza and drinking coffee at night, and I had a conversation with two girls from a wing. And there was a sharp cry and very loud breathing above me [there was a bunk bed in the room]. I was still sleepy, but I realised it wasn't a coincidence that Putin grinned in his speech. He did it. The war in Europe in 2022. The year 2022. The first thing I thought about was Dnipro, Sonya's relatives whom she's been trying to persuade to leave the city for some time. I had no money on my account to call her, and I was very scared to call. It's scary to inform somebody that the war has started and the cities are being bombed. It's like telling someone of the death of somebody close. I texted Max, and he called her. She asked me to come. I cried all morning, I brushed my teeth, and my salty tears mixed with toothpaste, I laced my Martens, and tears rolled down my skin, I walked through the collegium corridor where people were crying as well. They were calling their relatives, and my tears were dripping on the ground. I was running to Sonya, and I didn't even know that they were already bombing Western Ukraine and my Frankivsk. I took her phone and realised that Frankivsk was bombed as well. I cannot express my feelings at that moment with human words. That was the moment when the far-away war that was always somewhere in Luhansk, Donetsk, or even Kyiv (sure not here) started for me. There is no more here or there, we or them. They are bombing everywhere. Ukraine is united, from Lviv to Luhansk.

DOI: 10.4324/9781003449096-12

I called my parents, they were afraid, their voice was trembling. Everyone had gotten this animal fear then. Dad sent me a photo from behind the window; a black cloud of smoke was visible even from our Pryvokzalna street, far away from the airport. How could the fucking Moscow hand reach even our quiet and forgotten Frankivsk? Just how? I will never fully realise it.

Everyone was very anxious that day and made emotional, abrupt decisions.

Somebody left, somebody instantly mobilised and started helping others, and somebody froze. [...]

11:42 p.m.

- It's Star shopping now [reference to Lil Peep's Star shopping] ... but I'm afraid to look at the sky.
- Be strong, brother.
- I think it's the first time I'm afraid in my life. I'm lying in the living room wincing at every fucking sound Coco makes. [sister's cat]
- The main thing is to make it to the morning.
- Right.
- And it will get easier.

February 24

[...] I'm in Lviv, and nothing upsets me more than the news about the air-raid siren in Ivano-Frankivsk. All my life is there, my mom, dad, Evelinka. If anything happens there, I have no idea how to protect them from bricks and glass. The other day, I was so upset: wet eyes, weak legs, the taste of metal in my mouth. I really wished to become this metal sheet to cover and protect them all, and the taste of blood, so metallic, came to my saliva. [...]

February 26
After 6 p.m.

I called my dad in the evening, and he let Evelinka talk to me. She told me: 'Nania, when are you coming?' Then my dad asked her where and why they were running. She said, 'To the underground, for the bomb not to touch the body. Putin is throwing the bombs.' She's four years old. Her voice is calm; she doesn't realise a lot. Perhaps, that's all there is to realise, though. Maybe, we do not understand any more than she does? Why does my little sister have to understand it? I'm literally fucking torn apart. [...]

March 3

[The day before it all started] I read an article about collective trauma and memory. There was a quote there: 'It's not the echo of bullets at the edge of forest. It is a swarm of silver bees on the way to the hive of our orchard' (A. Mackus). This image of the silver bees was very intense. Reading that article, I didn't think I would live next to this image the next day.

I hate honey, and I hate the bees. I particularly hate the silver ones now.

I'm tired of being shocked. No more tears left. I don't know the way to break the russian propaganda mechanism.

Hearing: I like electronic music. It has little triggers, and it's emotional at the same time; it can be light, aggressive, and stylish. I do a lot of stuff while it's playing. It has a lot of broken, abrupt, metal sounds. Now, I can't listen to it. I don't know when I'll be able to. Every sound reminds me of an air-raid siren, a hit, a missile whistling, and once it comes to 130 bpm and 1.5-hour track, it's self-torture. I tried. I can't.

March 4
1:56 p.m.

The night was disturbing. We lay in bed, kept silent, and crossed our fingers for another way bigger Chornobyl not to happen [the occupants started shelling Zaporizhzhia nuclear power plant]. I started thinking: when would it be best to be born if I could choose the time? How would I experience this all if I was 12, 40, or 7 [years old]? [...] somehow, abruptly and hard, we found ourselves in a historical spiral, or even in its epicentre.

Touch: I spent 2 minutes in a hot shower today. It's a record. It used to be 40–60 seconds because of the fear of the air-raid siren and the inability to reach the shelter from the 4th floor. Hot water and intermittent breathing, the body is trying to relax, but I feel agitated, and my legs are weak because of this contrast, which gives me the creeps. I usually spend an hour in the shower. I'm really looking forward to when two minutes will turn into a nice, safe, and pleasant hour. For me, the shower is the ritual of cleaning myself from all that happened to me during the day. I always delay it until the last moment to get as 'dirty' as possible to then get as 'clean' as possible. This ritual has been interrupted as of now. And there is much more 'dirt' now. How long will I have to stay in the shower after all this is over?

Student space at K2
10 p.m.

[...] I've always tried to spend as little time at collegium as possible [but now it] gives me the strength to hold on. Maybe, it's just an illusion, a fear of exiting the UCU community right now, but maybe, I'm really looking at the community from another perspective. Grief unites.

March 5
3:25 a.m.

If the nuclear war starts, everyone will be fucked. Everyone is everyone, not just you. It calms down. [...]

I'm still afraid. I'm ashamed of [wanting] to go somewhere where there is no war. People are dying for me, and I want to flee. I haven't even heard the explosions next to me, just air-raid sirens. Physically, I can escape the war, but I can't escape it in my mind. I JUST WANT US ALL TO SIMPLY LIVE, as it's always been. And it's so hard to realise that it won't be as it used to be. [...]

Smell: There was a smell of pastry in the collegium today: a sweet, sugary, and a bit nauseating smell of pastry. The girls bake for soldiers, refugees, and volunteers. Such a smell should be at home, where it's warm, safe, and mom is doing something in the kitchen. Then she calls you, and you understand it's cookies or a cake by the smell beyond the kitchen door. [...]

March 6
5:25 a.m.

My chest is burning, it's difficult to breathe. I'm tired as fuck. Annoying questions never leave my mind. I can't control or suppress them. Who am I? What if I die not with the right people around, not in the right place?

Who are the right people? What is the right place? [...]

9:58 p.m.

Today, at a meeting with the team writing war diaries, Kolesnyk spoke about the body's vulnerability and its great strength. I agreed with him.

It was the first time in 10 days that I visited the centre, and I saw, even touched, the sculptures and facades wrapped in plastic tape and whatnot. Is this protection good enough against "Grad," shelling, fire, and shock waves? I don't think so. But it is important to people; they protect their own and will not allow anyone to own it. The city is as vulnerable as the body. It must be protected so that the body has a place to walk and live in later. [...]

March 10
2:47 a.m.

I'm sitting in a bathroom with my parents and little sister. Air-raid sirens have been wailing for 10 minutes straight. It's scary to listen to their nervous and intermittent breathing. At the collegium in the bunker, everyone's trying to distract themselves somehow. Here, there is silence, breathing, darkness, and this air-raid siren. The town is small, and one can hear all of them. The siren echo builds itself up. It's been a couple of days without the sirens. One gets used to good things quickly. I was overwhelmed by the last siren, as if it was the first one. [...]

The maternity hospital in Mariupol... Damn, did they hold a contest of the most beastly deeds there? Each new atrocity is worse than the last one. It was the last straw today. I want to believe it, but my gut tells me that they are capable of something many times, ten times worse.

Chemical weapons, for example. More precisely, 'we will apply it against ourselves', right? I have a deep burning in the right side of my chest. The legs are weak; breathing is hard. Back pain is partly solved, but a new one is coming to replace it. The body does not want to accept the reality we've been living for the last 14 days. [...]

March 11
12:15 a.m.

[...] It took the city too little time to calm down after the morning explosions. People have adapted to the war. Their rhythm and routine calmed me down as well. I realised that I'm mostly afraid of two things right now. I'm afraid of nuclear and chemical weapons and the catastrophe on one of the [nuclear power plants]. I more or less understand the way to act in such cases, and I keep repeating the algorithm to myself. But I don't want to. I don't want it to happen. I'm afraid worse things await us. I really want to believe in the best, but my mind has its own ways. I think these were all trifles, they've been playing with us, teasing us, but real disaster is still upcoming. If my life is threatened too much, I'll leave. But what distance from life to death will be acceptable to me tomorrow? And the next day? I don't know.

[...] It's strange. Uncanny. Unheimlich. And all the rest of the words of this kind. I keep delaying the moment to rethink death. It's time, I think. I'm not trying to accept it, it's unreal. I'm talking about being able to think about it freely, as the brain (instinct of self-preservation) blocks everything connected to it.

March 12
05:30 a.m.

Air-raid siren, 5 a.m. Managed to sleep an hour. I think it's the first time I had a dream. Two dreams. In the first one, I was sitting in the doctor's waiting room, but it looked like my room. I lived there when I didn't want to live in my main house. Once, I noticed that something was wrong. One of my paintings changed its position. I've never put it that way. And my photo disappeared. It was clear, the doctor wished me harm. I started packing my stuff from this waiting room-room and then realised that he had closed me there. I looked at the glass door of his office and saw him slyly smiling with one corner of his mouth, as I was anxiously jerking the handle. It stopped. I was sitting in the same room again. My photo was where it should be. But it wasn't in the right position again. The doctor stroked my hand and invited me to an exhibition and a dinner with some artists at his place. I accepted the invitation. I have bad eyesight in real life, but I always see well in dreams. It was the first dream where I didn't see well. I came to this meeting, and I saw a painting very similar to my own there. I shouted something, and the whole hall fell silent and looked at me. The doctor smiled slyly and said, "Oh, you did come." He looked at my hands all evening, and he asked strange questions. I woke up.

When I dream of something bad and wake up from it, I know clearly that it's not the end, it's always the series. Even if I tell myself not to sleep anymore, I will still fall asleep, and this paralysing horror always returns with a new plot.

In the next dream, dad was playing with Evelinka on the rug in the fireplace room. He squeezed her legs too hard with his legs. Her legs were getting blue and bled. My mother and I stood there crying, "What are you doing?" He continued to do it. The legs were all blue and covered with blood.

The doctor and dad are the people I trust, they help me, they wish me best. But in these dreams, they hurt me, and I'm afraid of them.

March 13

Today they showed us that no one can relax. Three hours on the bathroom floor. Earth and glass vibrating. 8 out of 30!!! missiles hit Yavoriv and one hit Frankivsk. I feel that I'm losing it, more and more with each air-raid siren. I can't make my close ones hide. Mom is very aggressive because she does not want to wake up the child 10 times a night. Dad breathes very loudly, intermittently, and he's losing it as well. I can't fucking take it anymore. [...]

March 15
12:29 a.m.

[...] I spent 5 hours sleeping on the bathroom floor yesterday. My body is in pain. I believe there'll be another air-raid siren in a couple of hours. Those bitches love nights.

Today, one of the applicants [for foreigners wanting to join the Ukrainian forces] texted this. I was in a relatively good mood, but when I saw this, I froze, it felt very cold, and my breathing went down to the belly. The brain pushes the truth away with the help of memes, Spring thoughts, patriotic mottos. And here's the truth:

> This is the last question i have for now, what will happen to our bodies if we were to fall in combat?

[...]

March 17
5:17 a.m.

I've got an impression that I lose some part of myself every day. How can we rebuild a place where 100 people died? How can you visit a "rebuilt" theatre if hundreds of people were buried alive in its basement? I imagined our Frankivsk theatre in Mariupol theatre's place. People are hiding under our theatre as well, many people. And this building is like a living being. It's like losing a close person. You walk there, pass this building all your life, sit on its stairs, enter it to see a play, look at it, love it, every day. How is it possible? I have no energy left. I just feel how it gets harder to breathe. I feel like a little powerless human. My legs and arms are weak and constantly trembling even when I think I am standing calmly. I'm very attached to my city, and the thought that it might be ruined suffocates me. I didn't start appreciating it more with the war; I always did so. I always enjoyed this quiet, peaceful city. I had these moments walking outside and willing to cry. I don't care if it sounds dramatic. Anyway, I won't forgive them for what they've done to other cities and hundreds of lives, but for my city, there's no fucking chance I will ever fucking forgive them at all. [...]

March 18
6:59 a.m.

Lviv airport. Fuck. We were so happy that it was the only one that wasn't hit. We were happy, and we were afraid about it. We were unwillingly waiting for it to happen, as it was impossible for them to leave it alone and to pretend it didn't exist. So many trips starting there, so many emotions since its opening, it was so new, glassy, stylish. Why? For fuck's sake, why?

Yurko heard the hit from his house a couple of km away from where it happened. I'm afraid for my friends, I hope they will calm down soon, and I will not break them mentally.

1:10 a.m.

Once I went to sleep after the air-raid siren was over (we had it simultaneously, Frankivsk and Lviv), I had a dream that I had to fly to

Istanbul with my dad. I'm afraid of flying, I'm so scared of it, and I always have such dreams. First, I was thrilled to go on a trip, but then I had a vision of our aeroplane being hit by a cruise missile. I saw an aeroplane salon on fire, screaming, and a second of weightlessness. All of it prior to this piece of metal falling to the ground from the height of 10 km and its second explosion. When I had this vision, I was looking at my full height in the mirror, and there was a suitcase under my feet that I was just starting to pack. I stopped doing it. I was very ashamed to tell my dad that I wasn't flying anywhere, and he shouldn't do that as well. He bought the tickets, the expensive ones, he worked a lot to earn money for it. He loves Istanbul. He's been waiting to go there. And now, he has to believe my visions, my freaking delusions? I squeezed a sentence out of myself, "I'm staying home." He packed his suitcase and went to the airport. The Lviv one. That was almost hit today.

Then I dreamed of an apartment that was actually an office. I came to give an interview to a man, but he just turned on the recorder, and we talked. He listened to me very attentively, took in my every word, looked very intently into my eyes and at my gestures. Then, my friends, classmates came, and he asked me to step aside. We went into a small corridor, and he told me that he couldn't take it anymore, that he missed his family, whom he had sent to a safer place. He started to cry, really hard. He leaned on my shoulder, even though he was twice my size, and I hugged him. He squeezed me hard; I felt his pain in this force. He cried so much, and the tears were so heavy that all my clothes were wet, as if I had come out of the sea. We returned to the room, and everyone asked me in surprise why I was swimming in my clothes … I stood motionless in front of them for about 2 minutes, and then I went to the mirror in the toilet. I saw that my eyes were covered with body plasticine. It was a kind of make-up. Everything from the eyebrow to the lower eyelid was covered with a bodily membrane. I don't know how I saw myself through it. […]

I have an impression that my body doesn't belong to me, that I don't make the decisions I believe to be making. I observe my hands, fingers, lips, nose, eyes, eyebrows, forehead closely. Who is it? What does it want and why is it doing what it's doing? I often have such splits, but they happen even more in stressful circumstances. […]

March 19

[…] Yesterday, I stroked my legs and arms and peered intently into the pores, microcracks, and uneven skin parts. I think I've never done it before. I didn't feel it immediately, as I usually do when I go from not noticing my body to being aware. I felt something warm and very close. I have never felt this with anyone before. It was a few minutes. And so, I see the marks of time and nerves on me, and I really want to get rid of them; I want to be fresh and vital, but I feel miserable, unattractive, I feel heaviness, greyness, flabbiness, dullness. [...]

March 23

It's heaven outside, so warm and lovely, I can't believe it. I was going back home and listening to Dakh Daughters. It's not the war that made me listen to them. It's been years since they joined my playlist. There's such strength and roots in what they are doing. I always get goosebumps. I miss my Lviv friends. I really need them next to me. When I see young people sitting on the benches or the café summer terraces, I see my friends and me instead. We are sitting, rolling cigarettes, drinking cider, and neighing so that the whole place can hear us ...

There were no sirens today, even the night was calm. It's great luck to be able to sleep well and not have to wake up. I thank the soldiers for this sleep and this warm, lovely Spring in my city. It's got too high a price, too fucking high a price. [...]

March 29

We were leaving Lviv to the sounds of sirens. There are many people at the railway station, some are hugging, some are waiting, some have already arrived, others are leaving. It's somehow very difficult and painful to look at, really fucking difficult and painful. At the border, the volunteers gave us water and food; they were very tired, but their sincere desire to help had not disappeared. We reached our point of destination easily and quickly (it could be much worse). When on our way, the E-siren went on,[1] and everyone was twitching. It's so that we don't forget why we are here. I love Kraków, and it hurts me to be here under such conditions and without my dad, with whom I often went here. Sonya's friend hosted us for the night. When I tried to sleep, I felt an intense burning in my chest, and it hurt to breathe. Every breath caused pain in the whole of my body. It never hurt me to breathe like that, except when I had bilateral pneumonia with complications. Neither a hot shower nor the absence of anxiety stopped this burning wave. [...]

March 30

We took train tickets to our village and went for a walk around the city. We walked in the centre, went up to Wawel, ate charlotte and a donut with chocolate and lemon. I got distracted, but along our route, many trigger points brought me back to peaceful times when my mind was clear.

The Poles are afraid; they are preparing bomb shelters and testing sirens. It's scary and bad, you run to a safe place, and a black cloud runs after you and breathes on your back. I was walking, and I constantly thought that it would be great if I were here with my parents and Evelinka.

Krakow is overcrowded. The sewage system cannot cope sometimes. I understand that such are the circumstances, that our people need to flee somewhere, and the local people are good, or they are also afraid (because the same thing can await them), and they cannot but help, and some sincerely want to. But I don't really want to hear our Russian or Ukrainian from every other person in Krakow. It disgusts me, it seems wrong that these people have to hang out here. I want Krakow with only Polish spoken and occasionally, very rarely, some other language.

April 7

From today, I don't want to write anything here. I don't see any reason to keep doing it. The war is way too long, and neither do I want to have a diary that is 'super long'. It will become a constant reminder of this fucked up, stretched-in-time, dirty, senseless war. [...]

Translated by Vitalii Pavliuk

Anna K.
March 2

On the morning of February 24, I heard a neighbour's voice through my sleep. She was talking quite loudly to someone. At first, I didn't understand why she spoke so loudly in the morning. But suddenly I had a dream again, in which I heard: "Anya, wake up! They started a war!" My neighbour's anxious voice woke me up. I did not believe what I heard. I realised that this is not a dream. [...] I felt panic. Because I began to realise how dangerous it is. [...]

I researched the map of bomb shelters. In the evening we heard a siren. We grabbed our backpacks and went to the basement. There were several children, a family, and two men in the basement. Next to me stood a girl and her mother. [...]

The thought came to my mind: 'Maybe it was a dream and there is no war?'. But of course, I understood that it was not a dream. It's just that when difficult moments come in life, you want it to be a dream. When my dad died, I thought it was a lie and a dream. But then I told myself that it was important to wake up, accept reality, act and try to protect Ukraine. From time to time, I asked God to save Ukraine, my family and the Armed Forces. I lived with a boy for five days. During these days, I kept in touch with my sister from Kharkiv. I was scared for her, because what I saw in the news was horrible. I did not recognize Kharkiv. I lived there three years ago ... I asked my sister to come to me and said I would help. She was afraid to get to the station because the Pavlovo Pole area was heavily bombed. She lived next door to Otakar Yarosh. The next day, her sister and her boyfriend decided to go to the train station and board a train to Lviv. For 21 hours they rode standing. Tired and frightened by what they saw and heard in Kharkiv, they waited for peace and quiet. My sister wrote to me that they were leaving, but they heard an explosion and the train stopped. It was the Muscovites who attacked the railway station in Kyiv. But after a while the train left for Lviv. I returned from the village to the apartment. I was a little scared to be alone in the apartment. But I told myself I was brave. A siren sounded at night. After the air alarm went off, I couldn't sleep, and my body shook a little. I tried to breathe slowly, but it didn't help. I decided to turn on the audio course 'Listen with the body' and started dancing [...].

During the dance, I turned into a seed that sprouted and stretched to the sun. The seed gradually grew and the tree grew. Fruits grew on me. I grew through the rain and the sun. The breeze enveloped me. I boldly moved to the sun to the music. I felt calm. The body no longer shook. I hugged myself and felt love for the world [...].

Translated by Victor Pushkar

Mariana H.
February 24

'Damn' was my first thought that morning. It all started with waking up at 7:00 a.m. I hate being woken up in the morning. I was in the UCU Collegium; my neighbours started shouting; they declared an emergency state throughout Ukraine. I read all the Telegram news channels and saw a message from my dad: 'There is a war in Ukraine'. [...]

February 25

I received a message that said there would be a shelling of Lviv at 2:00 a.m.; I did not unpack my alert backpacks. I decided to take a shower and wash my head before going to the shelter. 6 girls for 1 shower; each one had a few minutes because it was scary. Sirens sounded everywhere. We checked the news 24/7; we stuck together. It was easier that way; we were afraid to stay alone; finally, I went to the post office, and I got there in time. We went to bed fully dressed; we washed with the door open; the siren-shelter-rejection-anxiety. Damn, is this a reality? I want to wake up, but it does not work out.

February 26

I'm afraid of all sounds, even my own alarm clock or too-loud laughter. I'm afraid to go to the shower, wash my head, cook buckwheat, go outside—sirens wail everywhere, alarm, you have to run, escape. Panic inside, a "poker face" outside. And everyone is tired of the words: "Everything is fine, I understand you."

February 27

It seems I lived the previous days on adrenaline only. Today, I began to fully understand what is happening. In place of adrenaline a total exhaustion came. I can't put myself in order; the usual routine has been replaced by the ritual of scrolling news. [...]

March 1

Helping is a sublimation of worries.
   People burn their russian and belarusian passports and birth certificates. They are ashamed of their country. And I feel ashamed that I can't help on a full scale on the front line. It seems to me I'm not doing enough; I'm going in circles: camouflage nets, letters, humanitarian aid, attacks on fakes, volunteering to help refugees. But is that enough? I should do more; I feel anxious.

March 2

Art therapy and good music helped me to relax. But then a wave of emotions got me; for the first time in 6 days, I cried. While I was quietly biting my hands that tasted of tears in the corner, my dad called. I disconnected. I won't let them hear me crying. You get used to the sound of the siren and the shelter, but you still can't get used to the state of anxiety and the feeling of helplessness in the face of war. [...]

March 4

[...] I always wonder how people show their care and feelings, how they stick together, even the smallest ones. I used to be sceptical of the community, but now it is the only thing that saves me.

At the same time, fatigue turns into hatred. At putin, russia, the russian language. I still feel the burnout: I am like a match that someone set on fire once and tries again, but it is already burned out. It is about to turn to ashes, fall apart and be almost impossible to pick up. [...]

March 6

[...] I painted icons. I feel sceptical about this, but I decided that it could be a good art therapy. At first, I relaxed, then everything started to rage, then fatigue came. It's like the stages of the war, but it is multiplied by 2 in a couple of hours. [...] people are dying there, and I'm drawing angels here. Again, the trauma of the survivor. [...]

March 7

People and chaos make me angry. I constantly want to sleep; 12 hours of sleep does not help to feel energetic. Vice versa. I break down; I feel like a cup from an old set that falls apart from sharp touches. [...]

March 10

For the first time in six months, I had a dream. I sat in Zelensky's office while he read something carefully. I thought he needed support like no one else. I couldn't think of anything better and decided to just give him a hug. He said I should leave because they were going to record his video address. I politely left. At that moment, I saw a crowd of extras coming into the office. "Why can't I be there?" I stood aside. Zelensky confidently said something to the camera, and suddenly russian military men with machine guns burst into the room. They shoot everywhere, at everyone, those bastards. While I fall to the ground to hide, the extras are petrified, and the president continues to read his address. Through my fingers, I notice that the faces of those murderers are not just faces but holograms. It seems that putin's face is superimposed on the face of each soldier; they either mix or overlap each other; it's scary. Like a large army of one man. Recently I learned that putin has doppelgangers. Maybe that's who they are? I'm trying to fight off the bullets; I don't know what to do ... "Good morning! Get up!! Polya leaves for Georgia." [...]

March 12

[...] The sister says she likes the sound of sirens; it sounds to her like the singing of whales. For whales, it is a way to confess love and establish mutual communication. And for us, it is a message of danger, an alarm signal. It's scary that for her, it's just the usual sound, like a melody on the phone. Although it's good that she's not worried about these sounds. For me, it's the biggest trigger right now. [...]

March 15

Today, I realised that I am afraid of silence. [...]
Oleh, my dad's colleague, was sent to war today. It's scary, although he seems not to be afraid at all. [...] Mom said we needed him alive, and his little 2-year-old daughter needed him even more. At that moment, big, probably three times bigger than me, Oleh showed some tears, which he hastily wiped so that no one could notice; "men don't cry, especially in the face of war." And I say that crying is a normal reaction; I don't care about gender.
[...] Swiping through stories on Instagram, I saw that Max, my former classmate, was looking for a combat vest. I called him via video chat. It turned out that he needed it himself; he was with the Armed Forces near Odessa. Max always had the image of a bad boy at school. No one ever took him seriously; all the stupid ideas in the classroom were his. [...] But now, my classmate, with whom I drank vodka and juice in the 9th grade on a trip to the Carpathians and sang Rihanna's old songs, defends our country. He grew up quickly, and it's still hard for me to realise his courage. He told me that he was catching looters, going to Zhytomyr to study tanks, and wanted to have a bulletproof vest because "he would not be able to defend Ukraine with his bare chest for a long time, no matter how much he wanted to." During our chat, I couldn't squeeze the words out of myself; my chest froze, and I couldn't breathe; I just agreed and listened carefully to him. [...]

March 19

Today, at the meeting on the diary project, I thought about understanding and feeling that you are a person. When things do not make sense, when everything becomes common; when you are ready to give others what you would never have given away before. The experience of common grief, mourning, and loneliness unites. The noise reminded me of the desire of a person to merge with someone, to feel one imaginary body. [...]

March 22

Today is so sunny. We were walking in the park when the alarm sounded; it seemed people didn't care; nobody ran to the shelter [...]. It seems I've already got used to the sound of sirens; it doesn't make me so anxious as before; I start to hear 'the song of whales' my sister talked about earlier. I rejected the worst thoughts and decided to live; let it be as it will be. I enjoyed the rays of sun on my face, the reflections in the lake, and, oddly enough, the people who had recently made me so mad.

March 25

My sister [had] a dream. A rocket or its debris fell close to our house; it burned a little, then stopped. They decided to go. They didn't know where to, but they had to. In a panic, they quickly started packing things; my mom could not find her shoes for a long time. [...]

March 28

[...] Bastya and Sonya are going abroad. In the evening, we had some wine, as we did before when there was no war. Then we slept in the shelter and heard those sirens in the middle of the night again. For some reason, I felt very sad and anxious. Maybe that was because all my friends were leaving, and I would leave too, who knows. [...]

March 30

Today, in the shelter, Father Volodymyr told us about his wife. He said he felt she was "the one". He had been dating a woman for four years before that, and then only after two months of dating, he asked her to marry him. I have always loved listening to these love stories; each is so special. People are my great love, and they are so unique that they make me tingle. Every meeting by coincidence is not accidental, and each time, I understand how wonderful life is. [...]

April 2

The sirens woke me up at 3 am; we slept 4 hours in the basement on the ground. In the morning, Solya woke me up; she came from Tern to pick up her things and go abroad. On the internship in Prague. I'm glad she will be safe and have a job; one needs to get distracted somehow.

The rain washes away all the dirt from the streets; the drops slowly fall down from the houses and form puddles. I saw a photo of rain washing away the blood of shot people from houses in Bucha. I don't know how people can return to such homes. Could those ruins be called home at all? [...]

April 5

At night, a siren sounded again; already standard timing at 23:00 and at 4:00 [...]. Again, I slept on the floor in the shelter. [...]

April 9

Sasha came from Kyiv; she brought a cat and a dog with her. We need to take the dog to Lodz for an elderly volunteer from France. By the way, that was my dad's daughter from the first marriage who gave him the dog; when he went to the anti-terrorist operation in 2014, Milka went to war too. And his daughter left for moscow. [...] I have to cancel all my plans; I feel chaos in my head. Sasha will sleep with a dog in a very spooky hotel, in some basement room overlooking the wall. But love will overcome darkness. [...]

Translated by Henyk Bieliakov

Yelyzaveta B.
February 24

It's printed in my memory forever: the bed was still warm with sleep, a few minutes to seven in the morning; there was a telephone call from my sister living in Warsaw. She and N. by my side, who woke up with the telephone call, said simultaneously: "The war has begun". [...] I was looking into the surprised eyes of the boy who had not only woken up for those few seconds during which he was reading the message in Telegram, but had grown ten or fifteen years or so older.

In half an hour we were already dressed, serious and ready to do something, though we didn't know what exactly we were supposed to do. I saw resoluteness in N.'s face when he was packing our things into a small backpack. I saw the same resoluteness in my face too when I was passing by the mirror. And that resoluteness instantly switched into an exact plan of action for the coming few hours: to take only the most necessary, the most convenient and tested things along, to put the documents into a separate folder on the top, to hold the cat tight, because it was scared of cars, not to switch off my telephone and to comment on every move if we happen to have to split. In any other situation, I would praise ourselves for resilience and lack of hysterical panic. But instead of panic, we were feeling shock and understanding that there was no time for fear or for speculation. It was only A. who was not worried. He shouted from the kitchen: "I'll have some coffee and a smoke first, then I'll be thinking about it.".

It is even funny: I remember the two of us sitting at the table the day before, having tea and thinking that this increased state of strain was much worse than any negative swing of things; nothing was going on, but everyone was feeling uncomfortable, not knowing what we should be preparing for. When the time came, there turned out to be nothing to prepare for; there were no available skills. All we could do was act with reference to the situation and recall all the recommendations ever heard or read. [...]

February 24–25

We didn't manage to go all together to Poland; we lacked just a few hours; a law had been adopted to forbid men aged 18–60 to leave the country.

We nodded to the frontiersman, turned around and went back to Lviv. [...]

When we went to bed, N. hugged me very tight. I hugged him very tight in response. It seems like we were saying something to one another, but I don't remember what exactly. [...]

Early in the morning we got in the car and started off in order to take me to Poland to my sister's and N.'s mother with three teenage children [going] to France. His dad went with us in order to take us to the border. [...]

March 2

[...] Love is stronger than fear.

* * *

[...] Anger is eating me from inside. I am afraid that the strain in all the muscles of my arms and legs (that is exactly the way I have always felt a panic attack approaching me) will be added by my sister and her husband, who are losing the passion they were burning with during the first week. [...]

March 4

For the first time in 9 days, my head is being pressed by inactivity.

The looping of the first day, February 24th, is over, and I am not feeling myself within one morning anymore. But there is a different loop now, an endless circle of the evening when I came to my sister. Warsaw has always been a strange city to me, a coldly clichéd place. In thinking about Warsaw, I have always recalled the monumentality and the chimerism of multistory houses, a present from the state that doesn't exist. I have always recalled bitter winds and the historical centre, which is too artificial in its urban development. I have always recalled the attacks of panic and alarm that got over me during my previous visit. To cut the long story short, my memories of Warsaw are not the best. Now I've got neither a desire nor a physical opportunity to do the city's sights, to study the itineraries or to memorise the turnings and the abbreviations amidst the single-type apartment blocks. Previously, there were no manifestations of the internal riot, there was no equivalent of the childish foot-stomping: I don't like it, I don't want it, in two days I will come back to Lviv. But now my internal riot is dictated by indifference to all the external, and by my psyche's incapability of focusing on what is not connected with the course of the war. [...]

March 8

N. and I have been talking a lot about music for the past few days. First, listening to music was impossible, because every song was the time we could spend on something more useful. Besides, we couldn't afford to relax and to amuse ourselves. Though, it was not even the moment of willingness or unwillingness: we couldn't listen to music physically.

But in the end, music gradually returned to the steady flow of news and video reports. First, with Kalush song, which was played during the breaks of the telethon, then once a day in the evening during a smoke break—"Spring" by Dakha Brakha, and everything became bolder and bolder, until finally we sat down with N. and M. and created a joint playlist with Ukrainian songs. [...]

For me, this playlist became another evidence of me not being alone, not just because it had been drawn up in joint effort. It became important to me because every little thought I'd ever had or could have in future, every little feeling to describe which I couldn't find the proper word—all this had been experienced and was transformed into art. The fact that all the worries, fears and pains voiced and chanted in Ukrainian gives me an opportunity to feel myself as *one of us* instead of feeling lonely and forgotten no matter how lonely I was feeling amidst the foreign country and language, amidst strange faces and strange spelling, no matter how lonely I was feeling at the table with the people who had grown me up.

* * *

Since I spent the first four days in the car with very limited opportunities, I wasn't feeling hungry or tired. The main assignment was to cross the border; therefore, all my efforts were accumulated for it to be fulfilled, whereas the body's needs were reduced to the minimum. There was no time to feel any discomfort. I ate because I had to, I drank because I had to, I got up to stretch my legs for my joints so as not to forget how to work. [...]

After I got to Warsaw, I spent the next few days living in accordance with the survival principles: no hunger, no tiredness, no pain. I smelled only basic smells and my brain was too lazy to capture those smells, forgetting about them at once. There being no hunger, there was no satiety. There being no tiredness, there was no energy.

During the last two or three days, the instinctive routine was followed by a new, unknown feeling of round-the-clock boredom. Sometimes boredom is accompanied by the feeling of guilt; sometimes it just exists in my body like a separate organ of sense. [...]

* * *

N. has just telephoned me. We talked and laughed a little bit via video connection. He showed me Thomas who feels totally as the king of the house and does what he wants. I couldn't restrain myself and started crying: because N's intonations sounded too familiar (it appears that if I can't hear them every day, there is a fear that I can forget what they sound like); because as far back as a week ago I was sitting on that white sofa, thinking that everything would be all right and that we wouldn't split; because none of us knows when we will see one another; because with every day of the war, there are fewer hopes for it to quickly end. [...]

March 9
(From a dream diary)

In my dream, I saw the non-existent basement of UCU: a huge hangar turned into a bomb shelter. Rows of mattresses on the floor, colourful blankets that belong to students and staff, and scattered personal belongings. The mattress of M. who is currently studying for a master's degree and is a volunteer at the UCU humanitarian aid headquarters almost 24/7 is next to mine. The bed of my boyfriend, who is not a UCU student, is beside mine. The dream begins as if from the middle of the action. I find myself next to M., who came from the street with a parcel from his mother. We unpack the parcel and sort useful things: toothpaste, brushes, some little things. In addition, M.'s mother gave him bright and fine-smelling tangerines and a small brown book by Sartre. At one point, we realise that Lviv is being bombed. We don't hear the sirens. There are no windows in the basement. But as it happens in a dream, it does not prevent us from seeing the bombs fall on the Ground Forces Academy, and a huge pillar of black smoke rises above the building. Collectively (as if I share my consciousness with all those around me), we understand that they will hit the UCU next, and we will be blocked under debris without an opportunity to get out. M. is sitting right behind me, and we curl up in each other's arms, like those two prehistoric animals found in one hole hiding from the great flood. I am covered with M.'s body, his arms, and his torso; my hair falls on my face, and I can't fix it because we are not allowed to move. We pretend to be dead, just in case the soldiers come in. I'm lying down, my shoulders ache from the awkward pose, but I see that my boyfriend is also hiding someone under him. I think that if some people dig us, like those animals, up after a while, they would understand wrongly: after all, logically, we should cover each other, not other people. I close my eyes and hear the walls begin to fall. I wake up in the middle of the night from the absolute silence of my Warsaw apartment.

Why tangerines? Perhaps in my 1st year in university, tangerines became my personal symbol of university life, happy New Year vacations, and close friends for whom I carried them in my pockets. I even have a tattoo with them.

March 15

I can't recognize my reflection in the mirror at all. I've spent a long time examining it; my reflection looks like a picture of an unknown girl on the Internet. I am frightened by how my ribs and shoulders are protruded. For the first time in my life, I think it's too much: I am too slim. What I look like is sharp corners, ribs, shoulders and elbows added by dark circles under my eyes. There are shades not only on my face but all over my body as if I myself were about to become a shade. I have become faded and darkened with nothing but eyes on my face: two jewels, also sharp and wicked. I want to hide away from my own looks, but there is no place to hide away. [...]

March 28
(From a dream diary)

Before the war. I saw this dream a long time ago, before the war. Probably, those were the first days of February. I then spent the night at N.'s and woke up beside him at 7 or 8 am. At 10 am, he had a work call, and I, with my dislike of morning getting-ups and a great love of sleep, fell asleep for about forty minutes while he had a call in another room.

In my dream, I sit in my apartment in Lviv, in a class on trauma studies, and there are 5 other people in the video call with me—several classmates and acquaintances from Kyiv and Kharkiv. I'm not at all surprised that somehow we have a joint class (although Mira from Kyiv is studying in another department, and Ro from Kharkiv graduated last year). I just listen to them very carefully, smile at some jokes, and write down the question. During the class, I look at my apartment as if I had not been there for a long time and absolutely familiar and routine things amaze me: paintings on the walls, a blanket on the sofa cushions, the colour of the walls in the kitchen. I listen to the speakers and think that after the class I would have to go downtown because I have a meeting in the "Alterkava" on Stefanyka street. I memorise what they say to retell everything N. later. At some point, Mira, who is speaking, falls silent as if the connection is lost, and I turn my attention to the screen. Ms. Khrystya Rutar, my professor, is trying to find out if the connection has been lost or if something else has happened, and I can only hear a very loud bang that someone in the video calls a blast. I immediately know what happened: a Russian nuclear attack. Therefore, Mira's window is flooded with bright light and a loud sound. I look up and out of the window—it's mid-spring outside; the trees are boldly green; the sun is shining; the air is warm, and the light is diffused—I see an explosion on the horizon; I see the heat rising. (Although, in real life, the houses are situated outside my window, and I cannot see the horizon). The light becomes more and more intense until it totally blinds me. And I think: this is the end; I wish it would end fast. The pressure inside my body grows as if I suddenly have too much oxygen, and I can burst at any moment like a balloon. And I also think: I'm already dead, we're all dead, we'll finally find out what's next, after the earthly life. Seconds pass; the pressure doesn't go down, I can't breathe, it's dark before my eyes, and I don't understand why it's so dark for so long. Perhaps the whole after-death thing will be like this: darkness and uncomfortable pressure in the chest. My last thought is how can I do without N., I have to find him.

I wake up abruptly, and for some time, I cannot breathe at all, feeling the phantom pressure in my abdomen and chest. Outside the window, the spring sun shines, the curtains are barely moving from the thin draft, and a cat sits on the windowsill and looks at birds or other cats on the street. I hear N. saying goodbye to his colleagues in the other room. I go out to him and warm my hands over a cup of coffee for a long time.

I forgot about that dream for two weeks until the training started in Lviv, and the cars with loudspeakers drove through the city, broadcasting the sounds of air alarms and rules of conduct. Then, walking in the thin rain, wrapped in a coat and scarf, on Kostya Levytskoho street, I waited for a traffic light to change, listening to the sounds of those training and recalled that dream.

On March 15, my class coincided with the first air raid alarm in Lviv, and it was as if I was back in that dream without the opportunity to wake up. I had the desire to go blind and burst like a balloon.

March 29

Today, N. asked me if I thought that we could fail to see one another for another year or even longer. Of course, I thought about it. This is the thought that permanently lives with me, but sometimes it gains momentum and sounds so convincing that I stiffen or even stop thinking. This thought, as well as a number of similar ones (when will I see the room where I grew up? Will I be able to hug Mom and Dad? When did I see Lviv last time? Was that really the last time?) always approaches me with ice-cold breath in the back of my head, blocking my lungs and taking my speech away from me.

Over all, I [feel speechless all the time] as if words were tapped from me like blood. I am shivering, freezing and fevering without words.

[Will] we recognize one another when we meet? [...] We both will be beaten and ruined. [...]

April 3

I wish I could survive this war and say that I haven't shed a tear, because it was inadvisable at that time, whereas some people are always feeling worse than I am. Therefore, I was holding on, because I couldn't afford that luxury: to burst out crying means to give in.

But the truth is that I do cry [...]

Bucha.
Fear.

This could have been me.

April 7

[...] [I]ntrusive thoughts manifest themselves in different ways, more often when I am asleep when my psyche, tired of everyday overload, surrenders its defensive emplacements. When I had the first night dream in early March: the pitch dark and N's voice as if I had just closed my eyes and as if he were talking by my side. I was not glad about that, because these sample night dreams were followed by true night dreams: realistic imaginable events and memories from the previous life, distinct in terms of details. I see night dreams of explosions less often but there is always no sound of those explosions. I am lucky to have never heard them and to have never felt my body vibrating. Sirens roar with no sound in my night dreams as well, as if my brain understood that all these air raid alarms I've heard in movies, in videos and in the news are not my true experience. Therefore, it doesn't reproduce them. [...]

Manifestations of anger and aggression due to no opportunity to physically do anything or to damage anything are best softened by imaginable pogroms. Before I go to sleep, I close my eyes and wait a while, imagining I am ruining, breaking, or destroying all I can imagine: furniture, walls, windows, and people. I've got no feeling of guilt when I imagine that someone else's ribs are cracking under my feet or that someone else's skull is being crushed; they are not human, they are not animals, they are not alive. They look like humans but inside they are all ammonia and brimstone; they are something demonic and eternally evil, dead and disgusting.

I've never been able to talk about hatred for someone, even when poking fun. But now it is hatred that I am thinking of. I've found out about myself the following: to be able to hate this way, one's got to be not only furious but very strong as well. I've got an endless and unprecedented stock of strength.

April 8

It's a kind of magic, but today Warsaw smells like Lviv in spring. The pouring rain is followed by bright sunshine, the ground is wet, and there are young and brave leaves on the trees. If I close my eyes and stop thinking, I can imagine I am walking somewhere near the Park of Culture or Stryiskyi Park accompanied by birds.

Among the everyday sounds that I am missing are the noise of the trams and the hum of paving stones under my feet. Even birds are singing in a foreign language here.

Translated by Mykhailo Tarapatov

Miia K.
March 6

The 11th day of the war. It feels like ages have passed.

I am sitting in a safe place in a safe city: Krakow, Poland.

I remember the beginning well enough.

Thursday, 7.00 a.m. Sleepwalking, I was watching a message on Instagram; then I heard Mom's saying: 'A war has begun'. It made me and my panic wake up. I clearly remember the sky from the window of my beloved's apartment: the grey sky was frowning. At that moment a thought struck my head: Lviv is being bombed. [...]

I am feeling angry, aggressive, scared and desperate. [...]

I swiftly packed up my backpack to find out that a person doesn't need a lot of things to go away. I didn't pack any suitcase alarm; it took me five minutes to pack all the necessary belongings. I even packed socks with dinosaurs; my boyfriend had the same. [...]

I am not afraid to get acquainted with new people or to perceive them like my loved ones for the coming period of life. I am not afraid to go without plans for the future. I am not afraid to quit my job. [...] What I am afraid of is that my plans are breaking off until tomorrow. I am afraid because I don't know what my parents and friends will be doing without me. [...]

I remember the way we were going: no music, there were only fairy-tales for the little Solia. I remember having a smoke with Martha. There was no talking at all. [...]

There was a queue to the gas station, each driver being given only 20 litres.

We fed the children with the sandwiches we'd made as far back as when we were staying with our parents. The adults didn't eat. The human body is capable of more than it seems to be: loss of appetite, loss of sleep, only the most necessary things that must be done to keep our bodies alive.

On the way to the border, we saw armour vehicles moving near Chervonohrad and I became even more scared.

In the queue for green cards I heard a young boy saying: "They have started forcing guys to go back to Ukraine". I couldn't believe my ears. I couldn't imagine that they had started to close down the border for men. I still hoped they would let us go through, because my [boyfriend] was a retired military [serviceman].

They can't separate him from his daughter he loves so much, can they?

It took us 20 minutes to wait on the border. I woke up every time our car was moving another few metres forward. I was holding his hand all the time and rubbing my frozen palms, hoping they would let him through.

In the morning he told me to go forward and ask if they would let him through.

I went forward, it being cold outside though it was not bothering me, came up to a man with a submachine-gun who was inspecting the cars and asked:

- Good morning! May I ask a question?
- Go ahead but quickly.
- Are men aged 18–60 allowed to pass through?
- No, they aren't.
- But if he is retired?
- No.

My heart sank. I thought to myself: let us turn around to go back to Lviv. [...] While Martha and her little daughter were leaving the car, he told us to change to his friend's car and said that he was going back. 'Are you sure?' He nodded in the affirmative.

It isn't hard to go abroad. It isn't hard to get about in a country if you can't speak their language well enough.

It is hard to watch a father paying farewell to his child, not knowing when he will see her again. It is hard to watch him smiling and restraining himself without showing sadness or tears.

It is hard to imagine what is going on inside of him while he is hugging his little daughter with one hand and holding my palm with another hand.

Crossing the border, we went to stay with his friend's husband. I wonder how well our bodies can get mobilised: not having driven the car for 6 years, she was driving for so long without eating; she was just drinking water and smoking. [...]

When we came to the hotel, I threw myself onto my bed and felt deathly tired. I hadn't eaten for two days. I hadn't slept for two days. I was just smoking. The stress was thrusting every millimetre of my body. [...]

March 13

Today I had a nightdream that I was lying in bed, watching a missile falling down on the ground. Despite the missile being very close, it landed with no explosion. I was lying in bed with a friend of mine who began to laugh. I asked her to shut up, knowing that Russian soldiers were coming to us. She laughed even louder. The soldiers came to us to understand we were alive. Then they forced us to put on zapping belts. I pretended to have more pain than I was actually feeling and shouted. The night dream ended.

When I rose from my bed, [I read] the news of the shelling and the explosions near Lviv. My heart sank. Panic-stricken, I started writing to my parents and friends. Scrolling the line down, I read that not the city itself had been shelled. It was Novo-Yavoriv and Ivano-Frankivsk again. [...]

Sitting on the Vistula bank, I am talking with a friend of mine who has been learning in Germany already for many years. I can see a seagull dropping its huge piece of food into the water and flying to the water over and over again to get it back. It's a wonderful life: seagulls are shouting, fighting for pieces of food, people are running, riding rovers, taking their children for a ride and walking their dogs. But I look like a mixture of chaos and pain, aware of my helplessness, fear and fatigue, sitting motionless on a bench over here as if being all alone amidst this motion of life [...]

March 20

I am drinking Cabernet Sauvignon mixed with syrup in order to forget that I am not feeling anything. It feels as if my body were becoming heavier and slowing down. It suddenly hurts me and I don't know where exactly. The aquarium is making a noise in the background while I am listening to a serial. I can hear it but am not listening. I am all alone with my grief and I've got no right to scream. [...]

March 24

I am drinking wine again, trying to mute myself. It hurts me somewhere deep inside: it's hard to find an apartment in Krakow; it's hard to be far away; it's hard to keep all this inside of me. I am buying a lot of cheese for my mother, knowing that she likes it very much. Am I really trying to buy it or just trying to prove to her that I love her? I am telling myself: I am strong and I am doing all right. But yesterday I burst out crying, seeing a photo in Instagram "when the war ends, I will hug my father". I'd had no time to hug my mother good-bye before going abroad. I don't know if I will ever be able to. Deep inside of me, I feel like a taut string that brands with accumulated tears, emotions, pain and strain. I am in no condition to answer all the messages, neither from work nor from my friends. It seems to me I am falling apart into atoms, because I can't even keep my nose above the water level. I've heard the third crisis is followed by apathy and fatigue. However, I don't really care about anything. In a short while, my body becomes seized with the pain I can't resist. [...]

April 21
Krakow, 4 a.m.

I am fed up with travelling, with moving on and with birds in the park: it's too loud and painful. The first day in Krakow was eerie: I am still waiting for the sirens to roar behind my window. I am still raising my shoulders higher to my ears (I wonder if they will grow to my ears with time passing by, creating new bends of my body). I am still alarmed and it hurts me. Panic-stricken, I am still pushing the news to my parents that 5 fighter aircrafts have flown from Byelorussia, it being done by impulse. [...]

These bloody birds are irritating me. They are singing in the trees so wonderfully and carelessly; this bloody quiet that is pinching me is pressing down on me like a press or a pile of books you put above in order to straighten out that notorious abstract in order to take it to the instructor who will just throw it aside and give me the score. [...]

Until Monday it seemed to me that everything was all right, that I was warm, that I was being hugged and that I was feeling quiet, penetrated by tenderness and even happiness. Until Monday it seemed to me that the conditions of war didn't very much fit me to feel happy. Until Monday everything seemed to me more or less ghostly and remote. After Monday my life broke down the way it had as far back as then, on February 24th. I've got to feel crises and to scrape myself off again. [...]

I am doing all right / I am doing all right / I am doing all right / I am doing all right / I am doing all right / I am doing all right / I am doing all right / I am doing all right/ I am doing all right/ I am doing all right / I am doing all right / I am doing all right / I am doing all right / I am doing all right / I am doing all right

I am safe / I am safe / I am safe / I am safe / I am safe / I am safe / I am safe / I am safe / I am safe / I am safe / I am safe / I am safe / I am safe / I am safe / I am safe / I am safe / I am safe / I am safe/ I am safe / I am safe / I am safe / I am safe / I am safe / I am safe / I am safe / I am safe / I am safe / I am safe / I am safe

I want to go home.

It hurts me to stay here without hugging.

I want to get isolated.

Sometimes I wake up in the condition like "Where am I? What am I? What century is it? What had happened before I went to sleep?" I hope that this two-month long piece of life is just a scary dream.

Easter is on Sunday. On Sunday my [dead] brother would have been 35. On Sunday I will be especially fearing for my loved ones. On Sunday I've got no right to go crazy.

On Saturday is our anniversary, my boyfriend's and mine. I've prepared a lot of presents: from books to banalities as if materially proving to him how much he weighs for me. If I were allowed, I would buy up all the cheese of the world in order to present it to Mom. If only it could save her from the war. If I could, I would give everything away.

By the way, I've been in therapy already for 5 years. So, I know it for sure: I can't change the events or influence them; all I can do is get adapted and analyse them.

Thus, having researched my defence reactions, I am sure: I will survive all that, too.

But why on earth does it hurt so much? [...]

Translated by Mykhailo Tarapatov

Oksana K.
(*From a dream diary*)
March 13–14

In my dream, I had to interview three people on zoom. Zelensky was the first one. I asked him if he slept, ate, and drank enough water. And if it was hard for him to be a sex symbol of the whole world. I overslept the second interview, and the third one was with Alina Pash.

March 28–29

In my dream, I organised a big party for my birthday. There were a lot of people, a big fat cake, and loud music. Someone asked me why I was unhappy after I had been very aggressive. I replied that it was because of the wrong people there. I couldn't invite whom I wanted because of the war.

Anastasiia K.
March 15

[...] [E]very night, checking all the chats and news channels, I try to do it as quickly as possible so as not to disturb my parents with the light from my phone. But it doesn't always work out, so I quarrelled with my dad. And that affected my morning mood. I suddenly felt low. But then I thought: "I'm alive. Isn't that the main thing now?" And I remembered: yes, that is the main thing. It made me happy, and I felt easy because I was alive. I have another great day to feel the cold with my fingertips, close my eyes to the hot sun and chat with the vendors at the small local market, which is so dear to my heart because I am at home. I stay in Kyiv, and I don't regret it at all because it is my home. Here I identify myself, feel, dream, and know I am helpful. [...]

Unfortunately, it was replaced by grief because of the night shelling of Kyiv, which suddenly woke me, my parents, and Aunt Katya up at five in the morning. This unexpected anxiety and the sounds of explosions interrupted already not a too deep and peaceful sleep. [...]

I love my life no matter what.

Translated by Genyk Bieliakov

Dana K.
March 3

We were asked to write in complete silence, with no distractions, but nowadays not many people have such an option.

I live now in Lviv on Zelena street next to the Prohul'anka park with 4 migrants from Kyiv, a dog and my boyfriend. I am sitting in the kitchen, Sonia and Eduard (Sonia's boyfriend) are upstairs. Pasha (Sonia's brother and a friend of her boyfriend) is downstairs in the next room. Illia, my boyfriend, is somewhere upstairs taking a shower. There is a candle and puer on the table, there are some sweets and products on the windowsill, which we will take with us to the bomb shelter in case of an air alarm. For breakfast I had granola with milk—these days it's our typical breakfast. Palo Santo (an aroma tree which is sacred in China) smells nice next to me, even though it's not lit on.

I am constantly receiving messages about the required volunteers or the need to share some info on the accommodation for the displaced people, so it's hard to write without any distractions.

[...] The first few days of the war were the hardest. I couldn't understand my emotions. It happens often that I don't follow what I feel and cannot show my emotions. But in this situation, at the beginning of the full-scale war, it was even helpful, because I wasn't panicking, but I still realised that if I don't follow or share my emotions for a long time, they can grow into a sudden outburst of anger and resentment.

[...] I was angry, and sometimes I directed my anger in the wrong way. And my anger was there, most probably, from the realisation that many people have to participate in a cruel game that they didn't want at all. And of course, there is my personal hate, that I have to adapt to someone's rules in this game.

During the first days, everyone was frightened in Lviv. Every time on the way to the bomb shelter we were anxious. Every sudden move, sound and even just the opening of the doors were scaring migrants from Kyiv (friends and friends of friends of my boyfriend came on the 2nd day after the attack). I was a wreck, I couldn't control it. [...]

Also, it was weird how after a while I became indifferent to the possible death. I cannot count all scenarios of death I created in my head, while on the first night we were going from the border looking for a safe city and spent a few hours in Yavoriv. I decided to imagine all possible scenarios in order to know how to react in each of the cases and tried to figure out if it was possible to run away or to make my death quick and less painful. I was imagining rockets, explosions, my suicide in case of possible rape or maybe killing the attacker. In a while, I got tired of thinking about all possible scenarios, and the fear of death totally disappeared. [...]

March 4

[...] In the chats of the culture studies, they asked again who is where and how it feels. Interestingly, it's worse not for those who stayed here, but for those who left. Those who left are exhausted morally. And those who stayed are exhausted physically. My flatmates from Lviv, when they left, also said that they felt bad. It's probably the worst feeling that exists: to feel super guilty. Personally, for me, this emotion is unbearable.

March 9

I start realising the situation differently now. Now I feel like I lack the passion I had in the beginning. I remember that I gave my cosy apartment at the Rynok square to the migrants from Kyiv, who are not even my close people. There was my atmosphere, my personal space, and now I am not sure whether I will come back there. [...]

March 12

I am extremely sad for Mariupol, for shootings, shelling and mined "green corridor" by the Russian side. I don't know how to express my emotions [...].

March 13

[...] My boyfriend decided not to go to the shelter, and I thought to go by myself. Then I realised, that if they are indeed going to bomb us, I will come back for him, or I will stay in the basement for a long time, while he is injured. So I took my things, I put on clothes, took out my laptop and sat behind the door and a wall which split the rooms. The smartest would probably be to sit under the stairs in the apartment because there are the strongest walls which could protect me. But who knows if the stairs are strong enough.

It's interesting how different my thoughts are from my life before the war. That's it. The alarm is off. We survived. [...]

(*From a dream diary*)

On March 12 or 13, I had a strange dream.

A shell flew through the window into our apartment on Zelena near Pohulyanka Park. Somehow, I took it in my arms and threw it on the bed. The shell looked like a rugby ball but with sharp edges.

I didn't know what to do with it, and I was worried someone might think I brought it here.

I took a sweater and tried to pick up a mine with it and take it out of the room (in reality, of course, I would have acted differently).

I walked a long way up the stairs, afraid to accidentally drop the shell.

Then I got into the forest. It looked like the one in Ryasne, where I used to live with my parents, not the one close to my home. Then I went into the field. There were children playing football and volleyball, so I went farther to put the shell away from the children. I found the bushes and decided to leave the shell there.

I calmed down.

Suddenly a bird flew up and swallowed the shell.

I was worried that the bird would explode in flight. After a while, I saw an explosion in the forest, and I thought it fell there and exploded. Then that bird flew up to me and said she just spat the shell out.

Unusual dream ...

March 14
18:46

Bunt (mine and my boyfriend's favourite bar) started working again.

The law was not yet forbidding such places to work, because bars and pubs are paying huge taxes and it's important to support business for both the Ukrainian economy and the wellbeing of people, who owe businesses.

Yes, I am going to get drunk. Not too much, and [just] for the sake of [it], I really want to live at least one evening of my previous life and forget about everything that's going on around. [...]

March 16
10:00–17:00
[At a self-defence school]

I was training today to use the Kalashnikov rifle and again did some classes on first medical aid. [...] I was invited to give an interview to Italian journalists from *Fam Magazine* and other magazines.

During my stories, they showed me a video of dead russians and asked me to comment on it. I didn't know how to react. I just said that these videos are usual for a Ukrainian person today and people see much worse videos with dead Ukrainians every day.

Also, they asked me and my sister a few times if we [were] partisans in a way as if they already [knew] that we [were], even though we denied that and said that we [were] learning only self-defence and hoped that these skills [wouldn't] be needed. [...]

March 17
00:30

The cops are ringing in the door. We have a camera outside the door so my boyfriend decided not to open it.

My neighbours now are 3 guys of the conscription age, who are afraid to go to the army. Before they thought of going into the army as volunteers, even though they were afraid. No one went in the end. Only from time to time were they discussing it and hesitating.

My boyfriend came into the room and turned off the light. I said that in case cops knock on our door, I will open it and say that I am alone in the flat.

He agreed. But they are still standing next to the door and listening to what's going on there.

The cops are on our floor.

I hugged my boyfriend and heard how much his heart was beating. It was incredibly loud and fast. [...]

What a weird night [...].

Recently I [...] was walking with an Italian guy in the city centre and met my friend on the way, who was also walking with a foreigner. It was a bit of a funny story because we introduced foreigners to each other and it looked as if we were walking our pets. Now a lot of people I know are walking with foreign journalists or photographers, it's probably a new trend. My friend said a few sentences about the foreigner and that we have to meet one day because I couldn't find time through all this time when we could just sit down or walk and talk. And then he said, as if by the way, that he was taken to the army. He has training on Saturday. They just called and notified him. [...]

March 23

Vika asked me whether they could stay overnight at our place again because the earliest train to Uzhgorod is at 3 at night [...].

Now she seems to me even more beautiful than before and her manners are so easy. I remembered how tender and calm she had always been. [...] In the beginning, I was writing down some thoughts, as if it was her, in this diary. I was writing about what I see outside the window, about her fear of [me], writing down her words. Also, I was writing about the war, but not really seriously, but recently she sent me some of my writings and said that I should write more often. The text about the war made her worried because it was written when none of us could even think that it would happen for real. I was also surprised because I don't remember writing about the beginning of the war, but the handwriting is definitely mine. [...] Here is one of the writings:

"15th of December 2021. Today it's cold. Winter. The war is starting ... They announce the safety measures at Rynok square. I bought some oranges and lemon for my lover because she got sick. I am not sure if it makes sense to treat her. Anyway, we all will die soon." [...]

April 1

[...] I woke up feeling weird because I was dreaming that all neighbouring buildings were hit by the rockets and they were falling one after another. Then Illia hugged me and said that he is happy to wake up next to me every morning and fall asleep, so I forgot the feeling I had in my dream. [...]

April 3
13:07

Fuuuuuuuuuuuuuuuck. What the fuck?

I saw photos from Kyiv and Mariupol. I saw many photos and I read a lot before, but now I somehow sobered up and checked them all again.

What happened to these people in their childhood, that they are so cruel? And what for? They must realise clearly that they are not saving anyone through violence, it's rather their personal desire for revenge.

My friend, who is now training in the army, wrote: "It's really scary. If one looks at more photos – it's possible to get crazy from what they are doing [...] I do not want courts and investigations. I just want revenge for these scums. We must murder all of them, so they couldn't have offspring."

And I am here thinking about whether Ukrainians will ever start talking to russians. I have just decided not to talk to another person who is not ashamed that he/she is from russia. I can only maintain contact with those who left russia and deny their belonging to russian nation. [...]

April 5
00:03

I feel fucked, and I even cannot cry to let it go. I do not understand where my tears disappeared and why it's pressuring me so much. [...]

April 11
23:57

[...] I fell asleep during the day because I felt like a vegetable since this morning.

When I woke up, it was hard to breathe and keep myself on my feet. I went outside at 21:20. Illia texted: "Where are you going?" I answered: "Just to breathe".

Now apparently many people from Mariupol do not have such an opportunity "to go out to breathe", because they were poisoned by the chemical weapon at the same time when I went out here to breathe some fresh air. [...]

April 25

[...] I had a high spirit and wanted to help everyone around, and then I felt really fucked up and I didn't want to help even myself. At some point, I wanted to jump from the window and only thought that it was super dumb to ruin Illia's life like that, and the lives of my family and such a death is very out of time, helped me. [...]

Translated by Tetiana Fedorchuk

Oleksandra P.
February 24

I woke up because my parents were talking loudly and running around the apartment. I looked at the clock; it was about 6:00 a.m. [...] I started reading messages [on my university groups] and just got scared. "Kyiv is being bombed. The war has started." [...] I sat on the sofa in silence and thought that maybe I was still asleep, and it was all a bad dream. But unfortunately, this is my reality now. There were sirens that day, but no one ran anywhere; people were still as if in a dream [...]. We were home all day, packed our bags, and prepared cat carriers. We were preparing for the worst ...

[...] I miss my usual, boring life.

Translated by Yulia Kulish

Anastasiia I.
February 27
(*From a dream diary*)

A very short dream. I open the top door of the refrigerator (a freezer), and there's a heap of dog noses. Cut off, black, still wet and cold, but not bloody.

March 6
Hideout.

This word is the best to describe my need for a basement. The sound of sirens lets me be alone because only I react to them here. It is too strange and painful to hear some usual, everyday conversations of your relatives, the stamping of little children's feet while sitting in the basement. And you sit there, shaking, trying to understand what you are afraid of. [...] This basement without a door is in the house, so I go past it several times a day. I stare into the abyss that engulfs me, waking memories of a totally different time. [...] This basement is no longer just a way to save my life but my Plato's cave. Sometimes I go down there alone, hearing no external signal, to go through 5 minutes of hatred, as in Orwell's 1984, or to weep over some small thing. I no longer control my emotions, so all I can do is protect my loved ones from them. [...]

March 9
Pain.

Today, I read the news about Mariupol. There is terrible shelling. They carry pregnant women on stretchers made of improvised materials. People have bloody faces. And eyes. Their eyes look nowhere, but even they look for their previous peaceful life. [...]

It seems I have cut veins on my arms, and I am bleeding all the time. So I go for a walk around the town, leaving a trail of drops after me; I drink tea while the blood from my veins drips on my knees; I hug the pillows, treacherously leaving inconspicuous spots on their backs. No one sees this blood; only I feel it. As if only I have these unhealed wounds. [...]

I feel guilty for laughing sometimes. I feel guilty for not doing enough to make everyone laugh. What right do I have to distract someone from the war when my people die there? My friends' relatives are in the hot spots, while I can touch mine with my fingers.

Yes, I don't hear sirens in the town, but they still wail in my head. I shudder at every passing car, the sound of which reminds me of the aeroplanes flying. And I'm not alone. All people are like this. As if it is some kind of collective illusion. [...]

March 22

[…] I realised I have been in a deep mourning for some time now. I have been in a real mourning for the future, which will definitely never be the way I imagined it (because now I'm really afraid to plan anything), and for the past too, which will never be the way it seemed to go on forever. After all, they just shot my past and future down. And now I have to live with this emptiness in my chest. I have to live with this hole, through which the wind sings and even rain drops; sometimes crumbs of food and other trash fall there, but nothing can fill it anymore because the loss is too vast. It has hit me.

April 25
(From a dream diary)

In my dream, I was on that roof from a dream about brothers with black hair again.

But now I'm alone. Absolutely lonely. I turn around. No one is there. There are no doors or stairs that I had climbed before. Only the endless roof and the landscape of dark grey tops of high-rise buildings. Heavy fog covers the sky so densely that even the sun is difficult to see, although I know for sure that it is a day.

And I'm standing. Barefoot, in a light pink dress on a pile of snow. And I'm not cold. It seems that the emptiness inside me blocked all other feelings, and filled even my veins, which I sometimes feel through my childish, pale skin.

My body is only ten years old.

I raise my hands and lower my head to them. Amazing. Snowflakes fall from the sky, and light, pink summer apple blossoms land on my wrists and start to melt.

I am so fascinated by this moment of their rebirth that I can't take my eyes off them. The longer I watch them, the more it seems to me that the petals of these flowers are, in fact, a part of me. And they all melt and melt.

I start crying. I do not know why. It's a pity they were melting on me, and I can't take my eyes off the beauty of their deaths.

Tears fall on my hands, right on those apple blossoms, and they instantly coagulate like blood, biting into my body and leaving marks similar to large cigarette burns.

Now my baby's body starts turning blue and transparent. I feel that these wounds are draining me of my strength and my life.

I stopped crying and lay down in the snow, feeling that I would soon be completely eaten up and taken away.

I take one last deep breath and exhale as slowly as I can. It seems I can live on this exhale for at least another day of my life. Even for an eternity.

Until I wake up.

April 26
Abyss

To this day, I have often described my mood swings: the moments of self-understanding changed to the days when I felt totally confused.

However, now I feel relative stability. The answer to "how are you?" is finally found.

I'm still in Spain.

I have good living conditions here. I have my bed, my room, and even my doctor, who monitors my health. This is my first trip abroad, except for Bulgaria, so the beauty of Spain impresses me very much. Everything is so majestic and beautiful here, and people are in no hurry. They seem to still have a whole life to live, so they slowly enjoy their days. Several times I thought: "What if a bomb hit this beautiful place? This fortress? Or this huge Museum of Science built in the shape of an eye?" None of the locals think of it. Of course, they don't think of it. And I don't want it to happen. When my sister and I walk around the city, I always notice loudspeakers that could sound like sirens. And they do not. They do not wail and frighten people but simply silently wait for something for a very long time. I want to cry because I am like a mad girl in the city who hears voices in her head and talks to them. [...]

But these are just my minor problems. I have no right to (and I can't) enjoy the beauty of the local streets while people are dying in my native Ukraine. From shelling, rape, dehydration, and horror. I feel very awkward living between these parallels, and it is impossible to forget about them. In my thoughts, I am still there, lying on the cold grass in Stryi Park, curled up in a ball. [...]

April 29
(*From a dream diary*)

I had a dream where I felt I was in the world of Skyrim but not as in a game but in reality.

Autumn is coming, and the leaves are fading. I am the owner of the travelling theatre troupe; I am responsible for the costumes in this troupe, and sometimes I play the Clown on stage. My band plays in the *del arte* style. We drove to a strange village and decided to spend the night there because the road to the city was still long. And here we can give a performance as well.

However, there is a strange atmosphere in this place. There are few villagers and many cats. And the strangest thing is that no one in the village knows its name. As if it does not exist. Instead of people, I can see only some dark streets. [...]

The sun is already going down. The actors of my theatre troupe go to sleep in the carts in which they rode. I walk around, checking the area for suspicious persons while looking for some materials for the scenery for future production.

Suddenly, I see traces of blood. Little drops that fell under my feet. I am horrified because I saw them just as I was on my way back. To my troupe. They always rehearse songs before going to bed (this is our custom), so I immediately think someone might have heard them and tried to harm them. I understand that I can barely stand up for myself, but every actor and actress is for me as my family, and I am ready to kill for them, so I always carry a dagger. For self-defence.

I run following the trail of drops, and they do not disappear. They just get bigger. The sun is down, so I can't even see anything around me. My breathing is so ragged from running that I start to choke, but I keep moving. The dagger in my hand is already covered in my sweat.

I am back. There is total silence. Only torches shine. I look in one cart. No one is there. The other one is empty too. The actors' clothes and personal belongings remain, but the actors are not there. Where are they?

I go to the third and last cart with fear. I open it. I take a look in. Corpses. They are all dead. Everyone has a throat cut. They are piled on top of each other. Like some old rags. My actors. One on top of another. My family. Dead.

There are no traces of struggle, so they have been killed in their sleep. They will go to paradise.

But who killed them? For what? Who did they bother?

I started screaming. My throat ached. Out of anger, I started scattering everything around, smashing, breaking to pieces. I was totally drowning in despair.

Translated by Genyk Bieliakov

Bohdan S.
February 24

[...] At 6 in the morning, Linik called us and told us in hysterics that everything had started. We got on the Internet and found out that cruise missiles are being fired all over the country and the enemy is entering the cities. It was a shock. However, Ksenia was waiting for news from the school, about whether the children will go to school or not.

Now I can no longer remember everything - the day consisted of fragments, anxiety and paralysis. My stomach hurt, I felt nauseous and I didn't want to eat.

In the morning, I tried to withdraw funds, but all the ATMs were occupied, and the shops were overcrowded. It was scary. We have neither money nor supplies, how can we survive? [...]

February 25

Ours are fighting back. It is impossible to withdraw money, people buy up and leave.

Friends from abroad are constantly writing, offering help or options to leave the country. We are confused, everyone is crying except the children.

We gathered in the office, but no one knows what to do – we decided to accept refugees.

I hardly slept at night, and at 5 in the morning the alarm started, and we all went to the basement which is our bomb shelter. [...]

February 27

[...] I wrote to everyone I know with a request to help make the "war diaries" project. They answer, and advise, I created a file.

February 28

[...] We have a team – Igor, myself and Natalka Ilchyshyn. We will start writing war diaries together with students. We will keep the digital front, this also works. I suffer all the time because I don't do much – in fact, I can't do anything. But I decided that my task is our students! [...]

March 3

We have been holding the defence for a week. The russians have not yet taken any large cities, but they are actively destroying them. Terrible bombings in Kharkiv, Chernihiv and Kyiv. [...]

I finally started writing a diary, together with the students. We created a chat in Telegram yesterday and now there are 44 participants, although they are mostly girls.

A journalist from Britain came (Polyakov brought her) – they write a report about Lviv, she lived in Grozny, and they wrote reports from Afghanistan and Syria. I talked to her for a long time and told her about Lviv and the history of Ukraine. And then she asked, will Dnipro be the next capital? I was a little shocked – I say "but we will not give up on Kyiv." And she says, "I saw the russian war, they will destroy everything." And I became anxious and fear again descended to the bottom of my stomach. [...]

March 4

[...] The euphoria of the resistance goes down a little, depression begins from the feeling that all this is for a long time. [...]

March 5

[...] At night, a group of 5 young people came to us [...] they were military volunteers. Adam from Australia is a man of Algerian origin who came to fight for our freedom. Harden with a British passport and Stephen are still very young, but they came for something. They took different equipment, backpacks, and clothes. [...] Students also came to record their stories. The boys became local stars: I don't know if they will have time to fight, but I would definitely never go to fight for another country. I don't want to fight for mine either, there is anger and I want to kill the occupier, but to fight? I don't like it.

The whole day my body is on a swing – there is euphoria, then a fall, then a rise – then a decline. I have the impression that I am in Chernihiv, not the people who are being killed there. I keep telling Ksenia to go further west, but she doesn't want to, she says that our home is here. She is probably afraid. [...]

[H]ope is constantly replaced by despair, and you want to run away somewhere further, but you can't run away from it – we will all fight. [...]

March 6

[...] The physics of feelings is complex – my head turns on thoughts that drive the state of "everything is doomed" and this is immediately reflected on the bodily level ... everything shrinks in me, my body starts to shake ... then I try to mentally analyse this pain in details, directing my attention, and little by little anxiety and pain disappear ... and just as you begin to fall asleep, some invisible thought in a fraction of a second throws anxiety and fear into your body and again in a circle ...

March 9

[...] From the worst today – the maternity hospital in Mariupol was bombed ... I would have given up, but the war has no word of surrender ... only fight to the end, despite the casualties ... terrible.

Reflections are tough and difficult to write, but I have to start ... I am not traumatised, but rather depressed, I have to get out of it ... [Ukrainian Catholic University] wants to resume studies, I have to return to a strange life ...

March 19

[...] The work with the students went well – first we meditated, and then we talked – mainly about loneliness, death, about the fact that thoughts constantly direct us to do something, but the focus on the body allows us to understand that we are all equally lonely and independent beings who just need a team ... I am writing this and thinking about how these people live in occupied Kherson ...

March 22

[I] spent the night in the radio shelter.

There was a sad story in the shelter – a woman came with her 13-year-old daughter, Tania and Nastia ... they travelled for a day from Zaporizhzhia ... the woman's phone went dead, and when she charged it, her daughter called her and said that her son/brother had died in the war. The boy's name was Vlad. Now they will go to bury their son and return to Lviv, because the woman is afraid that none of her three children will survive ... panic, fear and pain ...

March 25

[...] I'm not fighting at the frontline, but I'm already dying [...]

March 29

[...] The predictions are bad – the orcs are forming a strong strike group and will try to capture Luhansk and Donetsk regions, gain a foothold in the occupied cities and hold the east and south ... for us this means another month of heavy war and a lot of loss of people and economy, cities and buildings and economy ... We won't get out of this shit even in 10 years ...

April 03

I woke up in the morning, but I didn't want to get up ...

Then as always the news feed and the horrible photos from Bucha and Irpin … headlines that this is the new Srebrenica, mass killings and rapes … violence against civilians … the orks deny everything and the Europeans are horrified … There is the disappointment that all this education, holocaust stories and mass murders do not teach anything, and the elites of the Western world think only about material things, especially the Hungarians – but we were also betrayed by the Georgians and Moldovans … there is a feeling that all this is for nothing … all this civilization … I want to run away into the forest and not deal with people …

The orcs are still gathering forces to attack Izum, which they have already captured … but it's all a complete disappointment … I can't look at these photos with corpses, these stories about mass rapes, about torn settlements … all this looks like in a bad movie … somehow I feel that it is a great blessing that we have a state that has survived, because if it was like Chechnya or like Ukraine in the past – all these mass murders would go unpunished … but there is hope for a tribunal, putler is an international terrorist and criminal, and his whole system is pure evil …

April 4

The night passed peacefully, although it was still dark when I woke up and I couldn't sleep … Ksiukha kept hitting something with her foot, she must be dreaming of something after that Bucha …

I went to work, trying to do something …

April 5

The war is still going on – the enemy wants to surround our troops in the east and gain a foothold in the south … People are discussing the text that came out on RIA, where the russians tell how they will de-Nazify and demilitarise us – it sounds like the doctrine that allowed the killing of peaceful people in Bucha and Borodianka […].

April 7

I woke up in a slightly melancholic state … It seems that the orcs are seriously advancing in the east and it is not known whether ours will be able to hold the territories …

April 18

The morning began with shelling – 5 rockets landed on Lviv, damaged the railway and bombed a tire firm … Rockets fly through Sykhiv … And at 11.00 the alarm started again […].

April 19

[...] I chatted with Matvii before going to sleep – he, like all teenagers, is shocked by the heroism of the defenders of Mariupol, their generation will have something to be proud of ... But I am worried that living in a state of war and being proud is not the best future for a child ...

April 20

It's hard to sleep, I dream of war ... My mind is waiting for an air alarm, although it falls asleep, it turns on at 5–6 o'clock and I can't calm down ... Mariupol, Azov, the dead are running through my head again and again ... I want to run away from all this [...].

April 22

I went to the Shroud to Dmytro in Ivan's church – it was beautiful and soulful ... He gave a sermon about the fact that Christ brought us to war - but this is a war with reassurance, salvation involves constant mental restlessness ... Constant war with oneself!

April 24

Today is Easter, so we packed up and went to Yavoriv ... There we took mom and dad and went to Lilia's ... We ate and drank, I said a prayer publicly for the first time, because no one wanted to do it ...

After dinner, Oleg came and we drank a little more, chatted, fried sausages... Nastia also came with her kid, they were walking the dog ... It is constantly raining, a true spring ...

April 27

[...] The enemy is pressing and advancing little by little into our territory, we are suffering losses and retreating ... War ... Everything is being destroyed around, Donbas will be a desert [...].

April 28

[...] In the morning I read disappointing forecasts about Kherson, the people there are brave, they are protesting, but it is not known when we will be able to liberate them ... But it will definitely happen [...].

May 1

It was warm and super cool, and the enemy didn't cause us any trouble ... We hung out a bit at home and went to the village, we also took Dania and grandma ...

I made a fire, did something, ate and drank, looked at the cherries ...

May 10

[...] In the evening we listened to Arestovych and Feigin – they all talked about the war, which is entering a difficult stage ... There is a lot of treachery around, people are spreading fear and it looks like a special operation in the digital world ... Difficult questions about Mariupol and Kherson, why the enemy passed through so easily in the South, why we have so many traitors ... I try not to read about betrayals because it is not the time, it is better to think about the future, but of course, it would be good if the guilty ones were punished ...

May 17

[...] Everyone predicts that the war will last a long time ... and this is frustrating ... In general, I'm tired of being Ukrainian, I want to become some kind of Canadian, without a family or a name [...].

May 25

[...] I try to convince myself that the loss of people, cities and territories does not mean the loss of the country, but every morning I wake up with the thought that we will lose this war, and there is no way out ...

May 27

Today we had the last discussion of the course at UCU, there were not many students – but we had an interesting talk ... Not everyone understands why to read Nietzsche, but it seems to me that now he is more relevant than ever – he was against nihilism ... Although maybe this is just my understanding of him because I am falling more and more into the grip of nihilism and do not want to embrace tragedy at all [...].

June 1

Today there was news about the death in the war of a teacher of the business school of UCU ... He was a very good man ... I once thought that if I was mobilised into the war, I probably wouldn't come back ... We have to prepare for the end, life may end ... Also today there was news from Zelen, that we have 100 people killed and 500 wounded every day ... This is only the military [...].

I'm preparing for a trip to the mountains, we have to go on Friday ... I've already filled up the car, I'll also take cereal and different things [...].

July 4

[...] Tomorrow the cabin will be delivered and the tea house will be installed ... Soon I will be able to spend the night in the village: silly dreams ... but maybe we will turn it into a micro-business and rent out the cabin to people who are looking for peace and comfort ...

Translate by Tetiana Fedorchuk

Annamaria T.
March 2
10:20 a.m.

Air raid alarm almost all over Ukraine. About half an hour.

Around 1 p.m.

our planes flew over. I heard them so loudly for the first time. My ears jammed, my heart pounded, my body began to shake, and tears came to my eyes. I am aware these are our planes, as there was no air force. However, the mind does not work at that moment, only the survival instinct. [...]

March 3
1:55 a.m.

First siren in the middle of the night. At first, I was dizzy, then I froze. However, the reaction did not change. They woke us up well. I was afraid we would not wake up. Now it's warm. The heart continues to pound.

2:51 p.m.

It's calm for now. I love to eat now, at least some break from this shit. Since morning, I have been weaving nets with Danya. My body, arms, and legs hurt terribly. I want to eat sweets all the time.

5:30 p.m.

Everything is fine for now. I feel tired all day. [...]

I cleaned up the living room a little, to feel useful at least somehow. They brought pizza here. Free food is always a nice idea. I began to appreciate my everyday life. I just want to get into a study routine and not be afraid of alarms. War really heals.

Ksu tells us about cats. She tries to teach us how to distinguish them. And I started to sneeze. Now is not the time to be sick. I hope it will pass.

10:10 p.m.

The first alarm of the whole day. We are worried about the invasion from the Belarus side. However, they refuse to attack. I hope Lviv will not be bombed. The city is beautiful, and it will be scary to live here.

Translated by Yulia Kulish

Daryna P.
March 3

The eighth day. My body is shaking at night after the sirens. I am not crying anymore but on the 2nd and on the 3rd days I was weeping wildly. [...]

Today I am dreadfully aggressive and I know that aggression is power-lessness. Apparently, my nervous system is already breaking down. My mother is eager to go abroad, my grandmother hasn't been sleeping for a week. She's been asking us to take her away, we are close to Belarus, and it is scary. [...] Today I am hysterical, having a huge feeling of shame for my imbecile behaviour.

All day I've been dipping into the telephone, looking through the news and social networking web-sites, reading other people's stories and watching videos with zombified Russians. I don't know why I've been watching it, it makes no sense at all. Watching it just demoralises and wears you [down]. [...]

While I was writing, I heard that NATO was not going to close down our sky anyway. So, they are standing on the side, watching us die. That's how it's going on! I was living just with one hope that they would close down our sky and we would stop being destroyed from the sky. I've got no more power to fight. I feel like howling. I am feeling very sad, because in a day I will apparently have to leave home. [...]

March 5

The tenth day of the war. Today I am feeling a little bit at ease. Two days have passed and I've been drowning in a sea of sorrow, apathy, etc. The emotional swing, such as aggression-sorrow-optimism is riding all day. But today I am feeling somewhat better. [...]

What I really want is to sing along with friends at a Ukrainian folk-art festival. On March 25th I would have to go to the mountains to participate in a training course for folk singers. I've been waiting for this event for so long but this is the way things have turned: the Orcs have spoiled everything, bastards. Now I am dreaming for it to end as soon as possible. [...]

March 6–8

The 11th, the 12th and the 13th days of the war were the days of derealization for me; I had too much internal aggression and my loved ones [were] suffering from it. Every day I have outbursts of aggression that fade away later. [...] [The] previous life no longer exists; it has disappeared and god knows if it will be the way it used to. This was getting over me on those days. I realised that the war and insecurity are going on at home, the previous life does not exist anymore. [...]

March 9

[...] It is surprising to me that at the time of war we find too many reasons to quarrel with our families but I think that's because our psyche is tired of nervous overload. We all are worried and the nerves are failing us. [...]

March 11

[...] This diary is a particle of my frontline. It takes me a lot of my emotional resource[s] to write about things needed here. My mind works very inefficiently and slowly; therefore, any kind of mental activity is very hard for me. I was mentally, emotionally and physically exhausted as far back as before the war. I got over the COVID infection exactly a year ago [but] I still have problems with cognitive activity. The Russia-Ukraine war and the stress it has caused makes my body feel even worse. It is still very hard for me to learn, think, express my viewpoint, speak foreign languages and pull myself together and in an adequate condition. [...]

March 15

[...] The feelings in the body brought by the war on its 20th day: tremor in the body and profuse sweating, worrying more than needed for small reasons and headache. [...]

March 16

[...] I am writing this diary at 3:15 p.m. By this time, I have already managed to feel a great emotional excitation accompanied by a kind of tremor in my body, as if I were jerked, and anxiety. [...]

It's 11:35 pm and I am eager to go to bed. Missiles from Belarus have hit Sarny, it's in Rivne Region very close to Lutsk. Provocations from Belarus have already taken place. Dad said it might be unquiet at nighttime. This is very scary and I am fearing for Dad and for my loved ones at home. I am very much afraid to go to bed, not knowing about the way the night will proceed. It is night that is the scariest thing at the time of the war. It's very mean: at night you are unprotected. [...]

April 3

[For a long time] I haven't [felt] so unwell like I do today. I am nauseating; I feel I am about to vomit with pain and non-acceptance. I won't endure it. I won't endure genocide of the Ukrainian nation. The poor kids are killed. Hostomel, Irpin, Bucha. Raped people are killed. What a big pain! I've got a dark dump pit, my heart is broken, I am being choked by the pain. Children! Forgive us! Please forgive us! We have failed to protect you! Oh, my god! It's just impossible to endure it! I just want to howl and scream and to get torn to pieces in this world! Russians were killing the civilians in Kyiv Region, torturing them and then burning down the bodies of the dead and running them over by tanks. I can't stand this pain anymore, it's impossible.

I can't learn though I need it badly. I can't pull myself together, my body is paralyzed. I don't know how to live with this pain; it's impossible, it's just impossible …

April 4

[…] There are too many thoughts. I am trying to carry on but there is too little reassurance around, the time is hard for everyone. We are working on it and if something gets over me today, I'll try to write about it here.

Translated by Mykhailo Tarapatov

Note

1 Translator's note: people have the app installed that goes on when the siren starts.

PART III

Resistance, Endurance, Testimony

8

UNEXPECTED SHAPES OF COURAGE

Emotions of Resistance in Ukraine

Marguerite La Caze

In addition to acting directly, experienced emotions can express resistance, and help to develop and spur resistance. This reflection considers how Ukrainians living under the Russian invasion have articulated the emotional upheaval and negotiated the effects experienced in relation to the disruption and horror of war. French philosopher Marc Crépon suggests that love and friendship counter and refuse violence and that belongs to the 'essence of life' (2016/2022, p. 4). Indeed, the Ukrainian authors of these diaries and dreams, writing soon after the invasion of their country on the 24th of February 2022, experience love, joy, gratitude, and hope, emotions that are linked to endurance, courage, confidence, and the will to survive. Olha K. writes that 'I can't help admiring people, I love everyone. Everyone who writes about being alive, everyone who helps, everyone who does something, hugs, calms down, sends music, news, cooks to eat, strokes a cat, goes to the pharmacy, takes photos, or saves lives [...] I love people and I am grateful for having many of them around' (March 1, p. 43). Solidarity with others also comes from the grief experienced in the face of loss; as Anastasiia B. says, 'Grief unites' (March 3), as grief is connected to love (Kelly Oliver, 2012, pp. 127–135).[1] The diaries and dream-memories act as a part of that process of countering violence—a care for the self that sustains the authors as individuals and as members of the community. Nevertheless, the feelings of desire for revenge, anger, and hatred, as well as courage and loyalty, can also play a sustaining role for resistors, as Lisa Tessman and other philosophers have argued (Tessman, 2005, pp. 116–125), and these are frequently articulated.

What is further evident in the diaries is that the authors feel they have to control their emotions of panic, hopelessness, and despair, or if not, hide

DOI: 10.4324/9781003449096-14

their expression from others, as these emotions are the most opposed to hope (Anthony Steinbock, 2007, pp. 440–450) and resistance. Their responses are in the moment, facing the uncertainty of what is ahead and incomplete, yet looking beyond the moment through this emotional resistance that builds courage. At the same time as experiencing the attack, each person is dealing with all the other emotional upheavals of their lives. One of the authors suggests that she is 'trying to describe the common feelings of all Ukrainians' (Khrystia M., March 2, p. 51) and while there is a wide variety of emotional expressions, there are common threads that emerge from the range.

Positive Emotions of Resistance

Courage is a classic virtue term, which can be unpacked in terms of its typical emotions. Like many such concepts, Western philosophical understanding of them traces back to Aristotle. He argued that courage or bravery is a kind of mean between excessive fear and excessive confidence. In the *Nicomachean Ethics* he describes courage as 'a mean with respect to things that inspire confidence or fear ... and it chooses or endures things because it is noble to do so' (1984 [350 BCE], 1116a10–12). Daniel Putnam suggests that 'Courage lies in the interface where the limits of our confidence meets the reality of a feared situation' (2001, p. 469). Finding courage means understanding the situation, in this circumstance the reality of war, and being able to act, and in Aristotle's terms, for an end that is noble. Mariana H. notes the courage of an old classmate who is in the army (March 15, p. 209). Anna K. admits that 'I was a little scared to be alone in the apartment. But I told myself I was brave' (March 2, p. 206). Telling oneself that is one way of making it true.

Tessman, building on Aristotle's framework, considers that courage is a virtue; however, given contexts of oppression, it is a virtue that can become a burden. In that case, while in one sense the virtue is valuable because it is aimed at liberation, in another sense it undermines flourishing as it does not contribute to well-being (2005, p. 125). She articulates the problem this way: 'the courageous disposition that the political resister is encouraged to cultivate in her/his character may crowd out other virtues in a deleterious way' (2005, p. 125). What Tessman has in mind is that aiming at courage could lead to a lack of appropriate fear, an insensitivity towards pain, an incapacity to experience emotions, or hesitance in forming attachments (2005, p. 126). Courage could lead to the sacrifice of the self, and in the context of war, frequently does. The burdens of courage have to be balanced with other emotions, and I argue that the diarists are able to do that through a range of means.

One way that emotions can be a form of resistance and build courage is through positive feelings and expression that support oneself and others. As Roger Gottlieb writes of Jewish people in the concentration camps of the Second World War, they 'saw everyday acts expressing the persistent choice of life against death. The Jews sang songs, wrote poems, dreamed of revenge and freedom and put forth the energy to share food, trade with one another, give support and love' (1988, p. 26). The diaries following the invasion of Ukraine also show resistance to the Russian propaganda. For example, Zhenia T. writes 'Russian propaganda like "why did u let Ukrainians kill Donbas people for 8 years?"' (March 24). The writers show compassion for each other and those displaced by the war, and this support undermines the views that Ukraine attempts to form 'an ethnically pure Ukrainian state' or that Ukraine forms a 'single whole' with Russia (Putin, 2021). As Timothy Snyder observes in his interview with Ezra Klein, the Ukrainian response to this propaganda is not a counter-myth or even a counter-history or narrative but is 'action directed towards the future', 'people who are engaged' and so building a collectivity through what they do and how they relate to each other, rather than through ethnicity or language (Klein, 2022).

For instance, love and joy are clearly and beautifully expressed in Olha K.'s entry quoted above, and such feelings of love are based on and create solidarity. In the first days after the invasion, the feelings were of 'panic, joy, anger, and anxiety' (Olha K., March 2, p. 44) but then sadness is experienced. Khrystia M. explains how emotional resistance can be understood: 'I can lead another front: to strengthen my spirit' (March 17). Those who are not in the armed forces have a part to play in maintaining their own morale and that of others. While there are feelings of fear too, they are balanced against the love. Miia K writes that 'I am afraid because I don't know what my parents and friends will be doing without me' (March 6, p. 219). Stefaniia K., says that 'There's nothing you can do about it, stay there and be afraid' (February 24, p. 59). However, Yelyzaveta B. says that 'Love is stronger than fear"(March 2, p. 213) and Mariana H. states that 'Love will overcome darkness' (April 9, p. 211). The writers express love for parents (Stefaniia K., March 6, p. 60), friends, and lovers. People also feel solidarity, as Yelyzaveta B. explains, 'The fact that all the worries, fears and pains voiced and chanted in Ukrainian gives me an opportunity to feel myself as *one of us* instead of feeling lonely and forgotten' (March 8, p. 214). Even though there is suffering, sharing it binds the community.

Mariana H. connects love of others and love of life, writing 'People are my great love, and they are so unique that they make me tingle. Every meeting by coincidence is not accidental, and each time, I understand how wonderful life is' (March 30, 2022, p. 211). Gottlieb noted that 'The greatness of Jewish resistors, lies not only in their courage, but in their capacity to call forth out of themselves ... a love of life, and of other people, and the capacity to manifest that love in a way which is both gloriously selfish and selfless at the same time' (1988, p. 37). As Anna K. describes, 'I hugged myself and felt love for the world' (March 2, p. 206). The diarists comfort family and friends, and feel a sense of belonging (Olha K., March 21, p. 47–48) and support (Stefaniia K., March 7, p. 60). Yelyzaveta B. makes that kind of comfort her mission: 'that was my role in this war: to remind people that they are important and that others remember them' (March 3). The Ukrainian authorities, led by President Volodymyr Zelensky, have continually stressed the need to offer each other comfort and express empathy (Bourke, 2023).

More simply, the authors also counter feelings of anger with those of enjoyment and pleasure, as Mariana H. explains: 'I enjoyed the rays of sun on my face, the reflections in the lake, and, oddly enough, the people who had recently made me so mad' (March 22, p. 210). They experience happiness or joy for many reasons: seeing loved ones (Stefaniia K. March 22, p. 61), feeling the sun (Anna K., March 2, p. 206), for resuming their studies and from teaching (Ihor K., March 10, 22, pp. 69, 70–71), hugging a friend (Ihor K., March 29, p. 72), for talking to her mother (Stefaniia K., March 4, p. 59) and just for being alive (Anastasiia K., March 15, p. 225). These experiences of happiness and joy are sustaining. Sometimes people feel relief: 'I'm so happy for her. Really, it's such a relief that someone I know is safe'. (Stefaniia K., March 3) and are pleased for others: 'I'm glad she will be safe and have a job' (Mariana H., April 2, p. 210).

Essential to living through the war is a sense of hope, expressed clearly by Mariana H. when she says that 'I hope nothing will fail, and we will have the strength to complete it' (April 5). Yelyzaveta B. has a will to survive (April 3, p. 217). Ihor K. feels 'A sense of healthy optimism' (March 1, p. 68). Fear is overcome in different ways. Stefaniia K. comments, as a number of the diarists do, that 'I feel like my fear went down. The initial panic has disappeared' (April 5, p. 62). Dana K., for example, calmed her fear by imagining many different scenarios of death (March 3, p. 226). However, for the authors, the experience of the war is so overwhelming that they may swing from hopeful and loving feelings to emotions of anxiety, anger, and grief in a single day. For example, Mariana H. writes that 'I felt better, but only for a couple of hours, then anxiety returned' (March 6, p. 208). So these complex feelings need to be considered, and I will reflect on the question of emotional swings further on.

While grief may be understood as a 'negative' emotion, the importance of grief in response to the loss of loved ones must be acknowledged. As I noted above, Oliver connects grief and love, and she makes this connection through the work of Robert Solomon, explaining why grief is morally obligatory as he maintained, and developing his ethical analysis of grief into a politics of grief. Grief can lead to a withdrawal in order to reflect as well as more active steps to respond to the loss, as Oliver notes (2012, p. 128). Furthermore, Solomon connects grief and gratitude, as we are grateful for the life of the one lost and our own life (2012, p. 130). The politics of grief that Oliver points to is one that extends beyond personal grief for close loved ones to concern about the value of life (2021, p. 133).

The phrase 'Grief unites' from Anastasiia B.'s diary, (March 4) is a very concise way of summing up how grief can function as a resistant emotion because it links those suffering in a group feeling solidarity with each other. In the context of the invasion, grief and mourning are complex, in that they are not only a response to a particular loved person but to the loss of the whole past life people in Ukraine had. Anastasiia I. writes: 'And then I realised I have been in deep mourning for some time now [...] future and past' (March 22, p. 234). Similarly, gratitude is not just for a single individual, although that is true too, but for the goodness of those who oppose the invasion: 'Goodness is quiet and imperceptible like air' (Anastasiia B., March 8). In contrast to these positive emotions that enable a resistance that keeps the authors engaged with the war effort, there are other emotions that make it difficult to mentally resist.

Undermining Emotions

One of the most expected responses to an unprovoked attack, anger, is also potentially debilitating. Zac Cogley argues that we can distinguish between virtuous and vicious anger in terms of its appraisal of wrongdoing, as motivation, and as communication (2014, p. 199). In his view, 'virtue can require great anger' (2014, p. 200). It is generally an emotional response to wrongs, injustices, and insults. For Cogley, anger is fitting or appropriate if a wrongdoing has been done and the anger is proportionate to the nature of the wrong.[2] He compares anger favourably to sadness and fear, contending that 'Anger has more beneficial motivational effects in that it moves angry people to engage with perceived wrongdoers' (2014, p. 209). He notes that anger does not necessarily lead to aggression or vengefulness, but it does mean that the appropriately angry person will be *'assertively resistant'* (2014, p. 211).[3] That resistance can be communicated in many ways. Notably, Cogley does not consider anger in response to war, yet his account could allow that retaliation is fitting as well as seeking other forms of resolution in the case of the war in Ukraine.

Thus, Russia's violation of the sovereignty of and invasion of Ukraine, and subsequent bombing of cities and attacks on civilians is appropriately met by great anger. Some of the authors experience anger (Mariana H., March 7, p. 208) and even rage (Mariana H., March 6, p. 208), and one could hardly deny that such feelings are fitting. However, Tessman's work alerts us to another two questions about anger. One concerns the possibility of misdirecting anger, and the other concerns its effect on wellbeing. While anger and even extreme anger might be the right way to feel in certain circumstances, such as when suffering under an unprovoked attack, it may not be the way to survive or to resist, especially over a long period of time, due to its corrosiveness (Tessman, 2005, p. 120). Tessman allows that moderate anger may not be the appropriate response; never-theless, we should not 'ignore how the resister is burdened by the imperative to carry an awesome level of anger' (2005, p. 121). Feeling what is the understandable and virtuous level of anger, a level that sustains resistance, can still mean suffering. For Tessman, that creates a dilemma between a moderate anger that is too accepting of injustice, and anger that is a developed response to that injustice, which could be all-consuming (2005, p. 125). To some extent, the authors take the second approach, so they can continue to resist. Ihor K. feels 'A lot of anger and tension in the body' (March 6, p. 68) but tries to become calm. Bohdana K. notes that she was angry for a wide variety of reasons at the beginning of the war, perhaps misdirected: 'my anger was there, most probably, from the realisation that many people have to participate in a cruel game that they did not want at all' (March 3).

Even more seriously, the authors fight against the exhaustion of hate as well as the corrosiveness of anger, as Olha K. admits: 'I'm tired of hating. Anger takes too much energy' (March 14, p. 46). While there is a desire for revenge, she agreed that 'aggression does not solve anything and that it is all too much' (Olha K., April 3, p. 49). Ihor K. makes the point that: 'Although I don't feel hatred now, I have no kind feelings either' (March 7, p. 69). Crépon argues that we need to ground a 'condemnation of violence and hatred' (2016/2022, p. 252). He allows that some wars may be just (2022, p. 241), although he does not mention defensive wars like that of Ukraine, but still avers that war must change our attitude towards death so that it becomes unacceptable. That change is both in the attitude towards the death of the enemy and in the sacrifice of one's own side (2016/2022, p. 244). It is hard to change these kinds of attitudes while being besieged, yet these comments show that even in this situation, the writers are reflecting on the questions that motivate Crépon.

In contrast, some of the entries describe sadness: Mariana H. observes that a man going off to war tries to hide his tears, but she believes that 'crying is a normal reaction' (March 15, p. 209). She also says that 'During the war, I never cried in front of people; I coped with everything inside of myself' (April 12). I will return to this issue of hiding feelings in the next section. Although there are problems for the resistant subject with anger, hatred, and sadness, despair must be the most undermining emotion that could be experienced. Anthony Steinbock argues that despair is what most deeply challenges hope, considering it in relation to similar experiences such as desperation, disappointment, hopelessness, and panic.[4] Referring to his own previous work, he defines hope thus: 'Specifically, the temporal orientation to the future was described as an awaiting-enduring (in contrast to expectation and possible impatience); the relation to otherness was characterised as a relation to some other-than-myself in the experience of dependence; possibility in hope was described in the modality of engagement and sustainability' (2007, p. 435). Some of the diarists could be described as experiencing expectation and impatience as they have a belief in victory. For instance, Yelyzaveta B. writes that the fear will dissipate 'because the victory will come' (March 3); and Dana K. states that 'I believe that I will survive and that we will win' (March 4). They are oriented towards a future where Ukraine is victorious, engaged in comforting others, and that helps to sustain them.

Interestingly, none of the diaries discuss desperation, although they do talk about panic. Steinbock thinks of panic as desperation without hope. A number of the authors mention feeling panicked, and they also discuss how they overcome that feeling. Anna K. writes that 'I felt panic. Because I began to realise how dangerous it is' (March 2, p. 206). To defeat panic, Ihor K. uses meditation practices (March 5) and Stefaniia K. uses a 'Don't cry, don't panic' written mantra (March 7, p. 60).

Steinbock then considers pessimism as contrasted to optimism rather than hope, because he sees hope as focused on an instance whereas pessimism is more general or applies to a sphere of life (2007, p. 440). Pessimism in that sense does not play a role in the diaries. However, hopelessness does. For Steinbock, hopelessness is 'the immediate and direct experience of the impossibility of the event *as* impossible', an event that I am invested in or engaged with and it 'projects itself into the future so that it closes down possibilities forever in this respect' (2007, pp. 442, 445). Ihor K. feels 'a sense of hopelessness, and my thoughts take on darker shades immediately' (March 8, p. 69). This sense follows the events of the war and the knowledge of friends and acquaintances in danger.

Finally, despair seems to pose the greatest risk on Steinbock's account. He says that despair is 'the experience of no recourse, no sustainability; every avenue is closed off. This absolute distance from the ground of hope is the experience of being abandoned, being alone, and being left to myself in the present' (2007, p. 449). The writers feel despair, but not constantly, and it often alternates with other emotions. Ruta R. mentions despair (March 3, 13, April 2, 11, 16, pp. 73–74, 75, 76) and helplessness (March 9, 16, p. 73) several times yet also makes jokes and talks about hope awakening (March 15, April 16, pp. 74, 76), and Olena C. also comments on her feelings of helplessness (March 6, p. 77) and despair (March 10, 13, 15, p. 77), but notes that her mood can change to euphoria (March 10, p. 77). Many of the diarists write about a 'seesaw' of emotions (Ihor K., March 13, p. 69; Olena C., March 10, p. 77), such as between euphoria and despair, and Dana K. talks about 'mood swings' between high spirits and lethargy (April 25). Such swings are one way that hope and hopelessness and hope and despair can co-exist as the diarists move between feeling that they can help everyone and that they themselves are helpless. Dana K. comments on these feelings, as well as the need to withdraw to reflect. As Hannah Arendt argues, for thinking 'withdrawal from the world is the only essential precondition' (1971, I, p. 78). This experience is clearly described by Dana K.: 'Mostly I think about everything in my head, and then I talk about the decision or one thought or an issue which appeared as a result' (April 25). Such thinking can help to resolve some of the seesawing as well as to make decisions.

Yet there are other emotions, such as guilt, that also make it difficult to cope with the experience of war. Dana K. observes that about those who left feeling guilty for leaving and that 'It's probably the worst feeling. Personally, for me, this emotion is unbearable' (March 4, p. 227). Guilt is also mentioned by Anastasiia I. (March 9, p. 233) and Ihor K. (March 1, p. 68), as is shame, by Anastasiia B. (March 5, p. 199) and Mariana H. (March 1, p. 207). The intensity of all these feelings is also balanced by control and secrecy.

Control and Hiding of Emotions

On numerous occasions, the authors describe controlling or suppressing their emotions, or hiding their expression from their loved ones. Mariana H. notes that 'The main thing is not to show fear to parents. I worry about them more than about myself' (February 26, p. 207). She hides the fact that she is crying from her father (March 2, p. 208). This concern for her parents demonstrates how Mariana H. is putting others first in her emotional life and considering how to alleviate her parents' concerns for her. She also refers to the sublimation of her worries through helping (March 1, p. 207). Stefaniia K. asks 'How can I even contain so much anxiety for others?' (February 28) while Olena C. writes: 'I just silently cried in the bathroom so no-one could hear me' (March 15, p. 77). Anastasiia I. speaks for many when she notes that 'I no longer control my emotions, so all I can do is protect my loved ones from them' (March 6, p. 233). Yelyzaveta B. considers how it is important to have self-control so that others can also do so (February 24, p. 212).

Other diarists find there is a blockage of emotions: Oksana H. reflects that

> I am in a strange condition ... well, on normal days I'm very, very much anxious. I feel anxious even when there are no specific reasons for it. In general, for any reason. I can just lie and feel anxious. After the war started, all my emotions have been kind of blocked, I don't feel anything. There is no fear, no aggression, no panic. I have never felt so calm. I'm afraid, when it's all over, all these emotions, which are now blocked, will return to me with new strength and I will have to deal with them somehow. (March 15, p. 79)

This response could be seen as a kind of self-protection; not to feel anxiety or other emotions is a way of coping with both the horrors of war and the everyday disappointments, like an air-raid alarm disrupting an English lesson, as it does for Oksana H. (March 15, p. 79).

Dana K. reflects on how suppression of emotions could have repercussions later: 'I still realised that if I don't follow or share my emotions for a long time, they can grow into a sudden outburst of anger or resentment. Later it indeed happened' (March 3, p. 226). She also says that 'everything is perceived [...] as if I were observing it as news from abroad' (March 28). Her concern about suppression is well-taken, but at the same time the capacity to exercise this kind of control shows everyone's agency and ability to resist. It is rare for the diaries to comment on resistance directly, but Kateryna L. sums up the complex pattern of emotion and resistance: 'They try to snatch the love of life from us with cruelty and tyranny. But the more pain they bring, the more the desire for life and resistance is generated' (March 1, p. 81). The writers are able to meet and counter the assaults on their lives.

Conclusion

While the diarists have different views about the purpose and value of keeping the journals, in a number of works, the self-analysis of emotions appears to act as a kind of resistance itself. Even though strong difficult emotions such as anger, hate, sadness and despair are experienced, they also find time for comfort, joy and love that enables their courage to take balanced forms. My short discussion cannot do justice to the full range of emotions and moods reflected on, such as pride, disbelief, shock, surprise, disgust, longing for the past life before the war, and apathy, so I have focused on those which are the most prevalent and form some level of commonality. Ihor K. reflects on the methodological principles for war diaries: 'accented experiences, interaction with various information channels, phenomenology, and experiences of living embodied people in the terrible times of war'

(April 8). His characterisation suggests some of the richness and significance of these accounts that describe with frankness the unexpected shapes that courage and resistance can take.

Notes

1 Ihor K. writes that 'Isolation and loneliness are what unites us' (March 19, p. 70).
2 Macalester Bell contends that appropriate anger is a way of opposing evil (2009, p. 178).
3 Emphasis in the original.
4 Steinbock characterises desperation as a last hope or the extreme of hope, where we try anything to make a difference (2007, pp. 437–439), whereas in despair 'one experiences the loss of a ground of hope as such' (2007, p. 446).

References

Arendt, H. (1971). *The life of the mind*. Harcourt Brace Jovanovich.

Aristotle. (1984 [350 BCE]). *The complete works of Aristotle*. Vol. I and II. J. Barnes (Ed.). Bollingen.

Bell, M. (2009). Anger, virtue, and oppression. In L. Tessman (Ed.), *Feminist ethics and social and political philosophy: Theorizing the non-ideal* (pp. 165–183). Springer.

Bourke, L. (2023, February 9). "It was amazing": Ukrainian journalist scores hug from Zelensky. *The Sydney Morning Herald*. https://www.smh.com.au/world/europe/it-was-amazing-ukrainian-journalist-scores-hug-from-zelensky-20230209-p5cj3i.html

Cogley, Z. (2014). A study of vicious and virtuous anger. In K. Timpe & C. A. Boyd (Eds.), *Virtues and their vices* (pp. 199–224). Oxford University Press.

Crépon, M. (2022). *The trial of hatred: An essay on the refusal of violence* (D. J. S. Cross & T. M. Williams, Trans.). Edinburgh University Press. (Original work published 2016)

Gottlieb, R. S. (1988). Remembrance and resistance: Philosophical and personal reflections on the Holocaust. *Social Theory and Practice, 14*(1), 25–40.

Klein, E. (Host). (2022, March 15). Interview with Timothy Snyder [Audio podcast episode]. In *The Ezra Klein Show, The New York Times*. https://www.nytimes.com/2022/03/15/podcasts/transcript-ezra-klein-interviews-timothy-snyder.html

Oliver, K. (2012). Robert Solomon and the ethics of grief and gratitude: Toward a politics of love. In K. Higgins & D. Sherman (Eds.), *Passion, death, and spirituality: The philosophy of Robert C. Solomon* (pp. 127–135). Springer.

Putin, V. (2021, July 12). *On the historical unity of Russians and Ukrainians*. Office of the President of Russia. http://www.en.kremlin.ru/events/president/news/66181

Putman, D. (2001). The emotions of courage. *Journal of Social Philosophy, 32*(4), 463–470.

Steinbock, A. (2007). The phenomenology of despair. *International Journal of Philosophical Studies, 15*(3), 435–451.

Tessman, L. (2005). *Burdened virtues: Virtue ethics for liberatory struggles*. Oxford University Press.

9

THE DETERMINATION TO RESIST

Dumky by Young Ukrainians

Luisa Passerini

I have been immersed in reading the diaries and dreams in *Diaries of War and Life* for days and days. Navigating this vast material brought to my mind a piece of music by Antonin Dvořák (1891), which alternates melancholic tones with cheerful notes, exactly like these writings do. That kind of music is called *dumky* in Ukrainian.

I find this reading inexhaustible and I lose myself in doing it. I re-emerge in order to write down some impressions and I get a feeble understanding of how costly and yet rewarding to write these pages must have been. Reading them is riveting and at the same time disquieting. It opens a complex world which is never accessible through the news from the media or the comments by critical analysts. These writings go beyond the usual purpose of a diary, recording daily life and creating traces of memory. The diaries are in themselves an act of resistance.

Diary Writing

The hybrid nature of diary-writing testifies to the existential value of this act. As the online advertising for Angela Hooks' (2020) *Diary as Literature* reminds us, 'blurring the lines between literary genres, diary writing can be considered a quasi-literary genre that offers insights into the lives of those we might have otherwise never discovered'. The decision to write is a way to interrupt the inexorable flow of small repetitive acts, the result of a choice to reflect on the flux of events and thoughts, a gesture of responsibility and appropriation of what's going on. It can be conceived of as a form of subjectivisation, through which the subject becomes more conscious of their situation and can question themselves on how to change it. Thus, it is a

DOI: 10.4324/9781003449096-15

courageous and somewhat risky act, even if it is induced by the request of a teacher in a protected area and with the prospect of a translation with an international resonance. 'I finally started writing a diary, together with the students. We created a chat in Telegram yesterday and now there are 44 participants', writes Bohdan S. (March 2, p. 237).

At the same time, writing is perceived like a privilege, although a difficult one: 'we were asked to write in complete silence, with no distractions, but nowadays, not many people have such an option' (Dana K., March 3, p. 226).

However, nothing is fixed and stable within a condition of war. While at a certain moment resisting requires writing, the context can change rapidly as time goes on: 'From today, I don't want to write anything here. [...] The war is too long, and neither [do] I want to have a diary that is "super long." It will become a constant reminder of this fucked up, stretched-in-time, dirty, senseless war' (Anastasiia B., April 7, p. 205). Here the resistance consists in the refusal to become a scribe of the war, a chronicler of something 'dirty and senseless'—because the very act of writing it down would seem like a legitimisation, it could mean transforming this dirty senseless thing into something meaningful, by ennobling and dignifying it.

The use of terms usually defined as vulgar or obscene (like 'fucked up' in the quotation above) reinforces the stigmatisation of the war (but let us not forget that 'fucked up' also means, according to the *Merriam-Webster Dictionary*, which classifies it under the category of 'vulgar slang', *confused, disordered, damaged*). The use of this and similar terms is recurrent in the testimonies of the War Diaries, sometimes in a censored form: 'what the f*** for [...] when all this bullshit started', 'some ***d-up shit', 'some f*** things'. Other terms, which would go almost unnoticed in daily reality, sound like a blow in the written form: 'Damn, it's been so long since I recorded a video' (Oksana H., p. 79).

In a war situation, the stress that 'damn' puts on the statement that follows it transmits a sense of irrevocability, underlining the unusual condition that has suggested this expression. Indeed, simple daily utterances and gestures are inserted into a tragic context, creating a dramatic mixture:

The war in Europe in 2022. The year 2022. [...] I cried all morning. I brushed my teeth, and my salty tears mixed with toothpaste, I laced my Martens, and tears rolled down my skin, I walked through the collegium corridor where people were crying as well. They were calling their relatives, and my tears were dripping on the ground. [...] Dad sent me a photo from behind the window; a black cloud of smoke was visible even from our Pryvokzalna street, far away from the airport. How could *the fucking Moscow hand* reach even our quiet and forgotten Frankivsk? (Anastasiia B., February 24, p. 196)[1]

'The war in Europe in 2022'. I remember hearing these words again and again during the first days of the war, when I went out of my home in Torino to do food shopping, in the bakery, at the butcher's. People would comment with amazement and alarm, expressing a not totally altruistic concern: 'Will it reach us?'. However, there was also a genuine worry about the war on European land, something unheard for a long time, since the Second World War, according to the people with whom I engaged in conversation. Yellow and blue flags were hanging everywhere, from windows and balconies.

In reality, there had been wars in Europe during the decades after 1945: in Greece, Czechoslovakia, Kosovo, to quote just a few examples. But collective memory—at least in Italy—seems not to have registered them as such, perhaps because these areas are perceived as peripheral to the Western part of the continent, with a very exclusive and elitist idea of 'Europe'. Everybody seemed to think that it would be sort of a *blitzkrieg* given the disparity of forces, but the war kept lasting. The radio, to which I listen every morning, counted the days of wars, at the beginning as if it were a matter of days before it ended, then more and more as an insistence on the unexpected situation—unexpected resistance, in various forms. Counting continued until it became absurd.

Diaries of War and Life shows a similar process. Counting days, counting hours, is a recurrent topos, signifying that the passing of time is painful and anguishing. Oksana H. records a mixture of sentiments: 'Good morning! This is the beginning of my war diaries. It is 9 a.m. sharp now. The twentieth day of the war. [...] 18:42, the second air alarm of the day, I'm sitting knitting and hoping to go out and to finish watching the cartoon' (p. 79).

Miia K.'s diary reproduces faithfully the hammering of the chain of days and news by starting with a simple list of dates:

February 24th

February 25th

February 26th

February 27th

February 28th

March 1st

March 2nd

March 3rd

March 4th

March 5th

March 6th

The 11th day of the war. It feels like ages have passed. I am sitting in a safe place in a safe city: Krakow, Poland. I remember the beginning well enough. Thursday, 07.00 a.m. Sleepwalking, I was watching the message in Instagram; then I heard Mom's saying: 'A war has begun'. It made me and my panic wake up. I clearly remember the sky from the window of my beloved's apartment: the grey sky was frowning. At that moment a thought struck my head: Lviv is being bombed. My boyfriend left the shower room, saying: 'To cut it short, baby: cities are being bombed'. (p. 219)

In a consummate literary style, Miia K. will inform us only at the end of her diary piece about one of the crucial elements of her state of mind: 'By the way, I have been in therapy already for 5 years. So, I know it for sure: I can't change the events or influence them; all I can do is get adapted and analyze them. Thus, having researched my defense reactions, I am sure: I will survive all that, too. But why on earth does it hurt so much?' (April 21, (p. 222).

Here is a very convincing description of internal resistance: having a clear notion of one's situation, recognising its gravity, and accepting the suffering it implies. In this case, the help of some sort of psychoanalytical treatment may have been relevant, but I don't think the strength of Miia K.'s statements comes only from this aspect of her experience. I believe that it rather comes from her coexistence with the thought of death, well before the war: 'Dad would often say: "I am not afraid to die, because I can die just once." I would nervously smile, knowing that when it happens, it will be too hard for me to recover from it. There are too many people I worry about. I remember how hard it was for me to recover from the death of my brother in 2015. I wish it never happened again' (March 6).

Recording her experience of death and mourning, Miia K. punctuates her diary with dates and hours:

Crocuses are already making their way through the ground in Krakow.

I've got a tradition to plan my boyfriend's mems in Telegram: 6 a.m., 12 p.m., 3 p.m., 6 p.m, and 9 p.m.

March 7th

March 8th

And some pages further on in the diary:

April 5th

You don't know how much it hurts to be alive.

April 6th

April 8th.

The diaries make evident that in war conditions the perception of time changes radically. Anastasiia B. writes: '10.03.2022, h 02.47 *even though it's a new day, it's a previous one for me, so consider it 09.03' (p. 199).

And Viktoria Y.: '[...] I realize that a whole week has passed. Up to a whole week. Only a week. Every single day stretches like a rubber band' (March 2, p. 83).

To be able to give words to the distortion of time, to name one's reaction to it, is another sign of resistance and at the same time a symptom of how difficult it is to resist: 'it seems that it will not end [...] everything looks like a confusion of many events and details' (Viktoria Y. March 2, p. 83).

This confusion is worded in the language of young people, which resonates all over the world with similar tones. We must know the references, otherwise our comprehension is too limited. When Anastasiia B. writes, on February 24 at 11:42 pm '[i]t's Star shopping now [...] but I am afraid to look at the sky. - Be strong, brother' (p. 197).

I have to look up on the internet to find out that the song by Lil Peep to which she refers, ends with this last stanza:

This music's the only thing keepin' the peace when I fall into pieces
Look at the sky tonight
All of the stars have a reason
A reason to shine, a reason like mine
And I'm fallin' to pieces
Look at the sky tonight
All of them stars have a reason.[2]

The lyric and the music give a sense of sharing—thus providing some protection, a brief consolation, a sort of safeguard—so that Anastasiia B. can conclude the day with a note of courage:

- The main thing is to make it to the morning.
- Right.
- And it will get easier (February 24, p. 197)

Music is important for inducing a sort of visual and corporeal memory, a memory of the body. The Ukrainian band Dakh Daughters re-creates for Anastasiia B. the time she spent with her Lviv friends: a group of young people sitting on the terrace of a café in the summer, 'rolling cigarettes, drinking cider, and neighing so that the whole place can hear us' (March 23, p. 204).

I feel deeply moved by this image of youth and their fleeting moments of joy. It is the image of a lost happiness or at least of a mindlessness that resists unhappiness.

In these narratives, the body is a recurrent topic. It is as if the war had made everybody acutely aware of the threat to their and others' bodies, for good or bad. In some instances, for good: 'Hugs have acquired a special significance now, they serve as an alternative language to transmit information, as therapy, and as mutual support' (Iryna B., p. 90).

But often for the worse with the experience of being split, body AND mind: 'I have an impression that my body doesn't belong to me, that I don't make the decisions I believe to be making. I observe my hands, fingers, lips, nose, eyes, eyebrows, forehead closely. Who is it? What does it want? ... ' (Anastasiia B., March 18, p. 203).

The body turns up in dreams too:

I wake up abruptly, and for some time, I cannot breathe at all, feeling the phantom pressure in my abdomen and chest. Outside the window, the spring sun shines, the curtains are barely moving from the thin draft, and a cat sits on the windowsill and looks at birds or other cats on the streets. I hear N. saying goodbye to his colleagues in the other room. I go out to him and warm my hands over a cup of coffee for a long time. (Yelyzaveta B., March 28, p. 217)

On the following day, as she realises that she cannot protect her own family from falling bricks and glass, Anastasiia B. expresses a desire for her body to become an inanimate object, sheltering her loved ones: 'My mom, dad, Evelinka [...] I really wished to become [a] metal sheet to cover and protect them all, and the taste of blood, so metallic, came to my saliva' (Anastasiia B., February 24, p. 197).

The transformation of the body into a sheet of metal emerges as a desire to protect others, but also to become herself invulnerable, insensitive, hard and unbendable. Like the 'metal sounds' of electronic music that she mentions three days later in her diary: 'broken, abrupt', 130 beats per minute, which is fast and vivace, but not extremely fast. Yet, for somebody under a war, 'it's self-torture' as 'every sound reminds me of an air-raid siren, a missile whistling [...]' (Anastasiia B., March 3, p. 198). And a week later: 'Today, at a meeting with the team writing war diaries, [K.] spoke about the body's vulnerability and its great strength. I agreed with him [...] and my body suffers so much. It is painful and embarrassing to tell someone about it' (March 6, p. 199).

Dream-work
Dream-work: The whole of the operations which transform the raw materials of the dream – bodily stimuli, day's residues, dream-thoughts – so as to produce the manifest dream. (Laplanche & Pontalis, 1973, p. 125)

Dreams have already appeared in Yelyzaveta B.'s diary at the end of the previous section of this essay, and in some way they are inseparable from diaries.

On March 12th or 13th, I had a strange dream. A shell flew through the window into our apartment on Zelena near Pohulyanka Park. Somehow, I took it in my arms and threw it on the bed (in reality, of course I would have acted differently) [... then she takes the shell in her arms and walks up the stairs ...] Then I got into the forest [...] Suddenly a bird flew up and swallowed the shell. I was worried that the bird would explode in flight. After a while, I saw an explosion in the forest. And I thought it fell there and exploded. Then the bird flew up to me and said she just spat the shell out. Unusual dream ... (Dana K., March 12, p. 227–228)

Here, resistance takes place in manifold ways: through the symbolic sublimation of war explosions; in the continuous exchange between lucid awareness and oneiric fablescape; in the feminisation of the bird, who becomes almost a reassuring girlfriend and acts out a happy ending. Dana K. adds two photographs to her writing: one of the shell and one of a flying bird. Suddenly, I notice a similarity with the ways of transmitting memory that I have studied while researching the memories of migrants to Europe, particularly for what concerns the relevance of the contribution of visuality to the oral and written forms of memory (Passerini, 2018).

Among the forms of resistance, a happy ending is perhaps the main difference between diaries and dreams: it is not possible in the former, while in the latter it makes sense and gives hope. However, the whole life during the war cancels the difference between waking and sleeping. What used to be wakefulness becomes a sort of nightmare: 'Today, while on duty at the volunteer headquarters, I talked with my friend about our plans after this nightmare, when we would *wake up* and win' (Viktoria Y., March 3, p. 83)[3]; 'I miss my usual, boring life' (Oleksandra P., February 24, p. 232); '[...] I can no longer stand the war. It's the second time when I dream of myself and my friend drinking at Kolos [...], and I literally drink one beer after another, and the time in a dream is the same as in real life' (Zhenia T., March 4, p. 54).

And what used to be the time of sleep is transformed into a period of nourishing desires that during the day seem impossible or unrealistic. Viktoria Y. continues: 'I want to hang out at festivals to the music of Ukrainian artists. I want to see Crimea. I want to meet the dawn on the railway'. All this becomes for her a sort of successful resistance to the nightmare: 'It really has quite a therapeutic effect; these thoughts give hope that everything will be okay, that this will be over' (March 3, p. 83).

Manifesting hope is the expression of full resistance, but it is also incessantly put at risk by the blows from reality: 'Today I woke up with the news about the attack on the Zaporizhzhia [Nuclear Power Plant] ... every day it gets harder and harder to open my eyes and get out of bed. Inside, there is only a feeling of emptiness, which absorbs more and more space' (March 4, p. 83–84). A few lines before, she had written that the reply to the question: 'how are you?' has now become: 'Woke up alive today [...] which means very little in peacetime' (March 2, p. 83).

Dreams are disturbed, as if chased out of the status of dream; awareness of daily life creeps in:

> For some reason, during the war, I learned how to discover that I was asleep in a dream. Before the war, I could do it too rarely and rather by accident. But now, when I am asleep I almost immediately know I am dreaming. I do not interfere in the run of action, but when things get too bad, when it becomes mentally difficult for me to live in a dream, I stop it. I also noticed that I either see dreams I have seen before, or I don't see anything at all. (Anastasiia I.)

Yelyzaveta B.:

> In my dream, I sit in my apartment in Lviv [...] I look up and out of the window—it's mid-spring outside; the trees are boldly green; the sun is shining; the air is warm, and the light is diffused—I see an explosion on the horizon; I see the heat rising. (Although, in real life, the houses are situated outside my window, and I cannot see the horizon). The light becomes more and more intense until it totally blinds me. And I think: this is the end; I wish it would end fast. The pressure inside my body grows as if I suddenly have too much oxygen, and I can burst at any moment like a balloon. And I also think: I'm already dead, we're all dead, we'll finally

find out what's next, after the earthly life. Seconds pass; the pressure doesn't go down, I can't breathe, it's dark before my eyes, and I don't understand why it's so dark for so long. Perhaps the whole after-death thing will be like this: darkness and uncomfortable pressure in the chest. (March 28, p. 216)

Of another of her dreams, Yelyzaveta B. writes: 'I saw the non-existent basement of UCU [University and College Union], a huge hangar turned into a bomb shelter. Rows of mattresses on the floor, colorful blankets that belong to students and staff, and scattered personal belongings' (March 9, p. 215).

This scene is exactly like what we in Western European countries like Italy have been seeing on TV and in newspaper photographs about the war in Ukraine. The overlapping of media images here and real events and experiences there has taken place, and yet there is an enormous physical distance between Yelyzaveta B. and us here. But she keeps cool, embracing her culture and memory to resist. In one of her dreams,

M.'s mother gave him bright and fine smelling tangerines and a small book by Sartre. [...] Why tangerines? Perhaps in my 1st year in university, tangerines became my personal symbol of university life, happy New Year vacations, and close friends for whom I carried them in my pockets. I even have a tattoo with them. (March 9, p. 215)

A tattoo inscribed in her own body, a body that carries bright tangerines to be offered to friends. I automatically remember Simone de Beauvoir's memoir, where she records when Sartre had the hallucination of being followed by *langoustines*. Yelyzaveta B. and I share something, across time and space. Emotionally, I feel close to her, although I am aware of the distance. But solidarity remains and strengthens the feeling that her resistance might receive new energy from my participation. It is a virtual participation, through writing—hers and mine—since writing too is virtual.

I remember vividly reading Charlotte Beradt's *The Third Reich of Dreams* (1966/1985). One of the aspects that struck me was the presence of the enemy in dreams of people she interviewed before the rise of the Reich. And I find this feature in the Ukrainian dreams as well. Sofia D.:

At the end of my dream, it was evening, and my mother and I had to set the table for some people. And when these people started to come, I realized that they were pro-Russian, and they began talking rot, some f***ing things. [...] And then, in the end, they started quarreling either among themselves or with someone else. And there was a church nearby, a very beautiful one, black, and gold, with high domes. Kind of gothic, somewhere between classic and gothic, and they started to destroy it, in short. And we literally ran from there to the car to leave. I watched how it all collapsed, how the domes fell, and how the water supply pipes began to flow up like a geyser, it was kind of close to the sea. Well, in short, all this turmoil. All these things. And we got into the car. There, I wrangled with someone all the time. And we left. But this was not a very pleasant feeling. (March 11)

And then some soldiers or policemen came and forced us to leave, lined us up and walked around for some reason, looking at us. And I really remember, I felt how tense my whole body was when I was standing at attention, because I was scared, I was trying to control myself and to stand straight. And I don't remember how it all ended. We were not shot and should be grateful even for that. (March 12, p. 66–67)

Charlotte Beradt also wrote of the premonitory nature of some dreams. Again, a recurrent feature for people under such threats: Anna K.: 'I recall I had a very interesting dream before the war … I was in the mountains with a friend. We tried to climb the ridge (it looked like Borzhavsky:))) And going up, we saw the nature burning all around. My friend said: "Anya, Ukraine is on fire". We ran higher up, but the fire followed us. We couldn't escape the fire, and I woke up' (recorded on March 30).

I have kept the worst dreams as last. Death and the dead populate them. Anastasiia I. dreams of being the manager of a theatre troupe and sometimes playing the clown on stage. And then she sees the actors of her troupe

[going] to sleep in the carts in which they rode. Suddenly, I see traces of blood. Little drops that fell under my feet. I am horrified […] I run following the trail of drops, and they do not disappear. They just get bigger. The sun is down, so I can't even see anything around me. My breathing is so ragged from running that I start to choke, but I keep moving. […]

I go to the third and last cart with fear. I open it. I take a look in. Corpses. They are all dead. Everyone has a throat cut. They are piled on top of each other. Like some old rags. My actors. One on top of another. My family. Dead. There are no traces of struggle, so they have been killed in their sleep. They will go to paradise.

But who killed them? For what? Who did they bother?

I started screaming. My throat ached. Out of anger, I started scattering everything around, smashing, breaking to pieces. I was totally drowning in despair. (p. 235–236)

Some dreams like this one (or the one by Anastasiia M. about her mother, April 9, p. 64) express total hopelessness. Other narrators alternate gloomy dreams about hostile and dangerous Russian women with pleasant scenes like this: 'In my dream, I saw a palace. Malachite walls with beet-colored fabric patches. And there were gold patterns on the walls. I was very comfortable there, better than at home and better than in my dreams' (Stefaniia K., April 17).

Rarely, but it happens, somebody dreams with humour, the greatest ever form of resistance. It reminds me of the role of 'daily resistance' that laughter at the dictatorship's expenses played under the Fascist regime in Italy (Passerini, 1984/1987, pp. 85–93). Antifascists who had experienced that oppression, like Piero Calamandrei (1889–1956), wrote about a 'moral' resistance (Calamandrei, 1954/2012), and historians who had acted as partisans struggling against Fascism coined the issue of 'morality in the Resistance' (Pavone, 2006). And the President of the Italian Republic, Sergio Mattarella, very recently (April 25, 2023) said that 'the Resistance was first of all a moral revolt[4] by patriots against Fascism for a national redemption'. So, there is a continuity, in spite of the deep differences, between the great historical Resistance against dictatorship and the small acts of resistance during everyday life, including minuscule acts of mockery. And dreams allow this type of light derision to emerge.

Oksana K. writes on March 13–14: 'In my dream, I had to interview three people on Zoom. Zelensky was the first one. I asked him if he slept, ate, and drank enough water. And if it was hard for him to be a sex symbol of the whole world. I overslept the second interview, and the third one was with Alina Pash'. Then, on March 28–29, 'In my dream, I organized a big party for my birthday. There were a lot of people, a big fat cake, and loud music. Someone asked me why I was unhappy after I had been very aggressive. I replied that it was because of the wrong people there. I couldn't invite whom I wanted because of the war' (p. 224). On April 13–14: 'In my dream, it was my wedding. It wasn't some guy I knew in real life'.

Alina Pash is a Ukrainian singer and rapper, who has launched on the WWW messages of solidarity to women wishing that her music can help women's future generations to discover the feminine power within. I learn from the Internet that she cuts the figure of a 'hooligan' (meaning somebody who breaks the system of worldwide spread stereotypes) in the context of Ukrainian Pop music:

Her music collides elements of R'n'B and Hip-Hop, intertwining them with facets of Carpathian ethnicities. Pash's live shows can be found on most continents of Earth, as she regularly performs solo concerts and takes part in major music festivals, including (but not limited to): 'Calvi On The Rocks', 'Electric Castle' etc. (Yabal, 2023)

It goes without saying that R'n'B stays for rock'n'roll. But I am interested in the hybridisation with Carpathian ethnicities. I listen to some of her pieces on YouTube: to her lyric video *Karpatska* (240.563 visualisations), of which I find only a bad English translation. However, the last stanza ends with a significant programmatic declaration: 'Listen good people to what I want to say: The time has now come to manage in a new way' (Pash, 2023). Under the auspices of this wish, my own writing can come to an end and I take leave from the Ukrainian *Dumky*.

Notes

1 Emphasis mine.
2 'Star Shopping', 2023. Emphasis mine.
3 Emphasis mine.
4 The revolt and the resistance can be 'moral'. Not the victory, as Jacqueline Rose has reminded us in her contribution to the special issue of the *London Review of Books* presenting a collection of responses to the war in Ukraine. Rose: 'In his 1940 essay, "Discussion of War Aims," the psychoanalyst D. W. Winnicott pleaded for a military but not a moral victory. "If we fight to exist," he wrote, "we do not thereby claim to be better than our enemies"' (2022).

References

Beradt, C. (1985). *The third Reich of dreams: The nightmares of a nation, 1933–39.* Aquarian Press. (Original published 1966)

Calamandrei, P. (2012, 26 April). *Il significato morale della Resistenza [Speech].* Passato e avvenire della Resistenza. (Speech given on February 28, 1954, at the Teatro Lirico in Milan) http://www.umbrialeft.it/approfondimenti/piero-calamandrei-significato-morale-della-resistenza

Dvořák, A. (1891). *Piano Trio No. 4 in e minor, Op. 90 (Dumky) [Musical score].*

Hooks, A.R. (Ed.). (2020). *Diary as literature: Through the lens of multiculturalism in America.* Vernon Press.

Laplanche, J. & Pontalis, J.-B. (1973). *The language of psychoanalysis* (D. Nicholson-Smith, Trans.). Norton & Co. (Original published in 1967)

Mattarella, S. (2023). "La Resistenza fu la rivolta morale dei patrioti". Speech on the anniversary of Italy's liberation from Nazi-Fascist (April 25, 1945). https://www.ansa.it/sito/notizie/topnews/2023/04/25/mattarella-la-resistenza-fu-la-rivolta-morale-dei-patrioti_95a0fc9f-2161-4c2d-84a5-d89b287fb2df.html

Pash, A. (2023). Karpatska [Song]. *Karpatska.* CHORNYY. https://www.youtube.com/watch?v=O6fb202ZGTM

Passerini, L. (1987). *Fascism in popular memory. The cultural experience of the Turin working class* (R. Lumley & J. Bloomfield, Trans.). Cambridge University Press. (Original published in 1984)

Passerini, L. (2018). *Conversations on visual memory.* European University Institute. http://hdl.handle.net/1814/60164.

Pavone, C. (2006). *Una guerra civile. Saggio storico sulla moralità nella Resistenza.* Bollati Boringhieri.

Rose, J. (2022, March 24). Day 5, Day 9, Day 16. Responses to the invasion of Ukraine. *The London Review of Books*, 44(6).

'Star Shopping'. (2023, August 21). *In Wikipedia.* https://it.wikipedia.org/wiki/Star_Shopping

Yabal (2023, September 09). *Alina Pash.* https://www.yabal.io/artists/alina-pash

10

TESTIMONY, ENDURANCE, *TRYVOGA*

A History Open to Shivering Bodies[1]

Magdalena Zolkos

Representing People[2]

The texts and images included in *Diaries of War and Life* offer their readers/ viewers representations of *a people*—people in the grip of violence, people experiencing fear, loss and grief, people 'shocked into action'[3] by the violence of war that they witness and endure, and people engaged in acts of resistance and defence. The question of *what kind of political people* Ukrainians have shown themselves to be in the face of the unprovoked invasion by Russia in 2022 has been asked by commentators and analysts alike.[4] Among others, Timothy Snyder in his influential analyses of the war has written and spoken at length about the Ukrainian *demos* that manifests through performative practices of citizenship, which centre on quotidian acts of solidarity, humanitarianism, and popular support for national defence. Referencing Ernest Renan's well-known formulation that 'the existence of a nation [is a] daily plebiscite' (1882/2018), Snyder has suggested that Ukraine's social mobilisation and resistance efforts should be interpreted as *an expression of political preference*—a kind of a 'vote' for national self-determination and political freedom—and thus as grounds for international recognition (Snyder, 2022). From this perspective, civic nationhood is 'not about getting its history in order', as Snyder put it in conversation with Ezra Klein (2022); rather, it consists of practical efforts of 'asserting [one's] own existence day to day' by a 'collectivity [that exists] because it is directed towards [a] future'.

The crux of Snyder's argument is that people emerge through resistance against imperialist and tyrannical power that threatens their political (and physical) existence, and that through their 'earnest struggle'—a phrase

DOI: 10.4324/9781003449096-16

Snyder borrows from the American abolitionist Fredrick Douglass—they affirm their freedom (Snyder, 2022). The struggle reveals the limits of tyrannical power not simply because it frustrates the military objectives of conquest (though that of course is also the case in Ukraine); rather, it becomes a *political event* insofar as the struggle casts into relief that in spite of all its destructive capacity, the aggressor is unable to quell people's desire for freedom. This imbricates closely with how the French philosopher of visuality Georges Didi-Huberman describes images of people rising in revolt against tyrannical power (2008/2018, 2016b). Through these images, Didi-Huberman argues (2008/2018, p. 64), we are afforded 'signals' or 'glimpses' into the fact that the work of destruction, no matter how horrific and calamitous, remains forever 'unaccomplished' and 'perpetually incomplete'. The relevance of Didi-Huberman's conceptual nexus between freedom struggle and what he calls, following Freud, 'the indestructible character of a desire' (2008/2018, p. 85) in the context contemporary of Ukraine is striking. As Bohdan Shumylovych also suggests in his contribution to this volume (referencing Didi-Huberman), the first-hand accounts of the war found in the diaries, dreams and images are akin to 'fireflies' appearing in the dark of the night. They are 'flashes' and 'intermittent light' that signal life, love and desire that survive the work of destruction, appearing *in spite of* and *against* the catastrophic horizon of war (Didi-Huberman, 2008/2018).[5] Snyder's performative conception of civic nationhood aligns then with Didi-Huberman's notion of uprising as the irrepressible impulse towards freedom expressed by images (and texts) produced in response to war and atrocity. In both accounts, the political people *appear* through acts of resistance against aggression that targets their political, cultural and physical existence (2013/2016a, p. 95).

The testimonies in *Diaries of War and Life* abound in narratives of people's input in the collective struggle against the invasion, and of daily expressions of kindness, generosity and bravery that demonstrate their capacity to withstand hardship and to stand in solidarity with others in these onerous circumstances. In this context, the feminist undertones of many of these narratives are also quite striking. They are visible in stories of 'minor acts' of resistance, many of which centre on care relations, including hospitality and hosting displaced people, sharing food and resources, volunteering and engaging in humanitarian relief efforts, producing camouflage nets, securing medical supplies, assisting foreign journalists, learning self-defence, etc. The relational aspect of these representations is apparent as people are frequently depicted being together and relating to each other; hosting and visiting, in conversations, seeing each other off to safety, welcoming and receiving others, cooking together, sharing food and booze, connecting on social media and in person, embracing, kissing, touching, making love and sheltering each other's bodies.[6] These 'minor acts' of resistance and the communal practices of care are both, in my view, performances of political people (in Snyder's sense) and an expression of 'people rising' in their 'indestructible desire' for freedom (Didi-Huberman, 2016b). At the same time, the relational care perspective also expands the notion of the people emerging in a struggle against invasion and unfreedom in that the diaries and dreams depict people not only *rising* (together), but also *holding* (one another). That relational orientation links the emergence of a political people to social care activities that, following Winnicott (1953), we could identify as 'holding environments' or 'holding spaces' created through quotidian efforts. Enduring war, together, means helping each other bear its burdens. It also means to *bear the unbearable*, bear the trauma of the war's violent imprints and ruins of the psychic and social life.

Nocturnal People

At the same time as the texts and images in *Diaries of War and Life* support and illustrate the notion that political people emerge through quotidian acts of defiance and struggle against invasion—and against conditions of unfreedom—these testimonies also point to the limits and perhaps even blindspots of an analysis that associates people solely with active subjecthood and with what I will call 'the diurnal domain' (cf. Bronfen, 2013). While these texts undoubtedly testify to the ways in which the threat posed by the invasion mobilised and activated the civil society and galvanised people into vigorous and (hyper) energetic modes of being and doing, they also offer glimpses into the 'nocturnal domain'— understood both literally (as that which goes on at night, in dreams, etc.) and as a metaphorical idiom for the dimensions of subjective life that come into visibility when people abstain from action and withdraw from the hustle and bustle of public life under conditions of war. Admittedly, these are often moments when stillness and inactivity are not desired or sought by the subjects voluntarily, but are imposed upon them; the withdrawal from activity can be enforced by the call to shelter (from air raids) and come from a demand put on the bodies to remain still in enclosed spaces. A substantial part of these testimonies consists of nuanced accounts of nocturnal life, including narratives and images of dreams, affects, fears, and desires. Writing of the diaries often goes at night as sleeping is repetitively interrupted by air alarms (see esp. Ihor K., *passim*). The spatial figuration of the 'nocturnal people' is their containment within the underground bomb shelter. It features in the dreams and diaries as a material container of human and animal bodies immobilised within it, waiting for the danger to pass (see e.g. Khrystia M., March 2, p. 51; Stefaniia K., March 11 & April 18, p. 61, 63).[7] Shelter is also a metaphor of a structure that is simultaneously protective and threatening as in Yelyzaveta B.'s dream when bombing turns the shelter into a mass of debris and transforms its shielding carapace into a tomb (March 06, p. 215).[8]

The 'nocturnal' designates those aspects of subjective life where consciousness loosens its grip on the subject: dreaming, fantasising, or intense affective experiences. Attending to this domain, and of relating it more closely to the political notion of the people, troubles the idealised notion of civicness as a social mobilisation and takes stock of the psycho-social costs of (hyper) activity and excitability induced by the conditions of war. The latter leads to depletion of energy, exhaustion, burnout and fatigue.[9] There is a recurring pendular dynamic in contributions to *Diaries of War and Life* as their characters move between active, diurnal life and its suspension or bracketing by moments of nocturnal withdrawal from activity, stillness and waiting. This peculiar war-time version of the Freudian 'fort-da' game ('now you see me, now you don't')[10] foregrounds a notion of the subject caught up in the oscillating movement between psychic, social and corporeal excitation and activity and the self's withdrawal from the public eye into a space of intense feelings, obsessive thoughts, the unconscious, and enforced stillness, where the traumatic effects on the psyche and the body become apparent (see also Frosh in this volume).

Centrifugal Voices

As figurations of political people, *Diaries of War and Life* affirms what Didi-Huberman calls the 'double difficulty', or 'double aporia', of representing 'a people' (2013/2016, p. 65). First, that difficulty is due to the fact that any attempts at grounding 'a people' in notions of oneness, coherence and indivisibility, even the people's coming together is the effect of the war is troubled by the irreducible plurality of views, affects, experiences and positions expressed in these diaries. Drawing on Hannah Arendt's discussion of kinship that, when incorporated into imaginaries of democratic togetherness, Arendt describes as a 'perversion of politics' (1993/2005, p. 94),[11] Didi-Huberman argues that the emergence of a political people involves plurality. He writes: '[politics] is interested precisely in [...] [those] *men*, whose multiplicity is modulated differently each time, whether it be in conflict or community' (Didi-Huberman, 2013/2016a, p. 65).[12] The second difficulty is that just as politics takes multiplicity and difference as conditions of possibility, the aesthetic field also deals with 'the fact of plurality' (Arendt, 1993/2005, p. 93). There is no singular or total 'image'; in fact, as Didi-Huberman argues, the word 'image' is a misnomer. There are only ever *images* 'whose very multiplicity [resists] synthesis' (Didi-Huberman, 2013/2016a, p. 65).

The political import of *Diaries of War and Life* is most apparent when its contributions do not comply with a uniform image of a unified nation. On numerous occasions the narrative and visual representations at hand resist the collation and homogenisation of peoples' experiences of war into an indivisible totality or 'oneness' of people who are united in their suffering. Instead, by asserting the irreducible *multiplicity* of positions, experiences and views, the diaries, dreams and images depict with unapologetic frankness subjectivities that *diverge from* the dominant representations of the war and of the civic mobilisation in response to it (including the recurrent homo-genising and idealising depictions in the West).[13]

An important part of such homogenised and unified representations concerns the domain of effect and emotions where certain ways of *feeling* are anticipated and approved, while others are ill-fitting and marginalised, so as to buttress the dominant representations of collective courage in the face of the war, moral superiority and victimhood. What is striking about the emotional depictions in *Diaries of War and Life* is precisely the extent to which many contributors resist and defy these hegemonic representations and expectations. With this, they refuse to gratify and be disciplined by the 'Western gaze' that exerts pressures on them to comply with these (often contradictory) representations: bravery in the face of war that manifests as an unfaltering will to fight, the outpouring of gratitude and thanks to states granting protection to refugees and offering military and humanitarian help, uncompromised social solidarity, etc. Examples of resisting these representations in the diaries abound, such as Anastasiia B.'s description of seeking protection in Krakow, in which she defies the frame of a grateful refugee and refuses to be reduced to victimised subject position. Characteristically succinct in her depiction of the host society, Anastasiia makes only two observations: she notes the palpable fear among Polish people as potential targets of a future attack and remarks on the quotidian difficulties caused by the influx of refugees, such as strains on the urban infrastructures and failures of the sewage system (March 30, p. 205). Pitting the physical reality of blocked toilets and the lingering stink against the infatuating narratives of Polish-Ukrainian kinship, the text resists discursive idealisation and stops in their tracks those readers who crave gratification for being 'on the right side of history'. Refusing the dominant norms of socially sanctioned behaviour and feelings (what emotions are 'appropriate' to the 'gravity' of war?), other authors also give a strikingly honest and non-idealistic account of a gamut of emotions, narrating ambivalence, annoyance, frustration, disillusionment even revulsion and disgust. They admit being reluctant towards participation in direct combat (Dana K., March 17, p. 229; Bohdan S., March 5, p. 238), frankly record failures of solidarity and support (such as instances of theft at train stations crowded with refugees), at times voice aversion towards humanitarian and volunteer work, and, on numerous occasions, express desire for revenge (e.g. Dana K., April 3, p. 230). Last but not least, they are unabashed in their representations of some of the Western responses to the war, calling out cases of ignorance, naivety and opportunism.

This quality of psychic honesty of the narratives and photographs extends to their representations of beauty, joy, and pleasure as 'things' that do not disappear during war, though they might 'clash' with some of its representations (see e.g. Dana K., March 14, p. 228; Khrystia M. March 2, p. 51; Anastasiia I., March 9, p. 233). These qualities are perhaps ever more important as they anchor the subject in life-nourishing and life-affirmative experiences and relations with others. A striking case of a critical response to censorship of aesthetics and feelings deemed 'incompatible' with the war situation is in Dana K.'s diary entry from March 14. She records being enraged at a German photographer who edits a sunset image to align it with the dominant iconography of war, thus toning down the photograph's colours for a 'dramatic effect'. 'To my mind [it is] almost the same as lying about the number of victims', Dana K. writes. And she asks: '[w]hy is it necessary to lie about the fact that there is beauty during the war [?]'. To use once more Didi-Huberman's words, the beauty is the sunset forms a 'rend' in the cultural aesthetics of war imagery; a 'suddenly manifested knot of an arborescence of associations or conflictual meanings' (1990/2005, p. 19) that needs to be thereby neutralised or removed. In contrast, the perspectives in *Diaries of War and Life* offer an assortment of dispersed and centrifugal voices that 'pull away' from the singular and unified image of a singular and indivisible 'people'. In his analysis of images from the Ringelblum Archive Didi-Huberman speaks of 'scattered ways of looking' and 'scattered moral perspectives' (2019, pp. 10, 16), making the point that resistance against oppressive power often takes the form of seemingly mundane and disconnected actions and gestures. They articulate political people in spite of (or because of) remaining 'plural, divided by breaches, fissures, conflicts' (2019, p. 38). *Diaries of War and Life* are precisely such representations of heterogeneous, disunified and 'scattered' people, who constitute a political community through relational practices of endurance.

The Trembling Subject

In the previous sections, I have suggested that the contributors to *Diaries of War and Life* articulate 'nocturnal people' by bringing into the field of visibility elements from outside of the ('diurnal') domain of active life, including the narration of secret fears, dread and anxiety; outlining dream-images; painstakingly mapping intense affective experiences. The significance of emotions and effects that can be further illuminated by situating these texts vis-à-vis Pierre Rosanvallon's taxonomy of democratic representation, which distinguishes between 'opinion-people', 'nation-people' and 'emotion-people' (1998). The 'opinion-people' (*le peuple-opinion*) highlights the effects of verbal articulations of positions and viewpoints for the formation of the democratic subject, and the 'nation-people' (*le peuple-nation*) focuses on cultural and political attributes that form the scaffolding of national identity. In the case of the 'emotion-people' (*le peuple-émotion*) collective political identity is expressed 'in a pathetic mode' (Rosanvallon cited in Didi-Huberman, 2013/2016a, p. 67). Drawing on that taxonomy of representing (and imagining) people, Didi-Huberman (who critiques Rosanvallon for his questioning of the democratic relevance of emotions) proposes that attention to feelings, effects and embodied sensations is key for opening critically the question of *who counts as a historical subject*. It is by paying attention to not only the quotidian, but, I argue, also to the nocturnal that historical subjectivity (and historical experience) can be pluralised beyond the dominant state-centric, masculine discourses of war and nationhood. In this context, the importance of the archive of *Diaries of War and Life* lies in their depiction of how people as (in Arlette Farge's words) 'beings of the flesh' become subjects of history; how they are 'acted upon' by history and, in turn, how they also 'act upon' the self (Farge, 2007, pp. 9–10, cited in Didi-Huberman, 2013/2016a, p. 77). These psycho-social records of war imbricate closely with a theoretical position according to which 'history is not recounted solely through a sequence of human actions but also through entire constellations of passions and emotions felt by the people', which 'opens history' to the presence of 'affected bodies' and 'affective bodies' (Didi-Huberman, 2013/2016a, pp. 77–78).

One way in which such affective history manifests in these texts is through the figure of a *shivering body*. A shivering, trembling body is neither moving nor static. In the diaries, the bodily shiver can come in the absence of means to verbalise an experience: 'I [feel speechless all the time] as if words were tapped from me like blood. I am shivering, freezing and fevering without words' (Yelyzaveta B., March 29, p. 217). Mariana H. writes: 'my hands tremble, and I start confusing words and merging several into one' (February 26, p. 207). The shiver varies in intensity and volatility. It registers on the body war's violence and as such it places the subject within the war's history as part of the political people affected by it. It is both in the present and in relation to the past and future:

> [M]y body is already shaking so much I just can't keep myself on my feet. And I wouldn't say that I was shaking with fear, no. If I was worried, I was most afraid [...] for the future of my country. Everything looked consistent in my head: there will be no country, no future for my people [...]. (Polina S., February 24, p. 88)[14]

The shivering body is not a diurnal subject—active, deliberate, controlling, balanced—but an unstable one, out of control, and, in a way, out of the bounds of their own body. Daryna P. confesses: '[there is] a kind of tremor in my body as if I [was] jerked' (March 16, p. 248), and Anastasiia B. notes: '[my] legs and arms are weak and constantly trembling even when I think I am standing calmly' (March 17, p. 202).

The shiver is a seismograph of the body in a shelter, thus separated from the proximity to the blast. It registers upon the cutaneous surface a quake (a bomb exploding) that happens elsewhere and at a different time. This is conspicuous in Stefaniia K.'s account of a shelter from April 18: '[w]ith somebody whimpering in the background, and with wehaveseenthemissilefromthewindow-itwassobig-therewassomuchsmoke, I felt the abominable creepy shiver in my stomach. The one that used to live in my guts in the first week [of the war]' (p. 63). For Kateryna L., the tremor is a point of connection between bodily interiority and exteriority:

I can't describe my thoughts at the moment when, already in bed, *I feel the earth tremble from an unknown shock.* And then, having found no signs of obvious danger around, I go back to bed, trying to calm *the heartbeat and tremors in my hands*, knowing that I'm falling asleep in a minefield, where anything can happen overnight. (February 27, p. 80)[15]

The shivering bodies in the Ukrainian war diaries *insist on being seen* as subjects of history in their distinct corporeal and affective experiences that form at the interstices of movement and stillness, but are not identical with either. A quiver, tremble, convulsion, tremor or vibration correspond neither to the representations of bodies in a frenzy of activities and movements nor to figurations of bodies that are immobilised and rendered powerless by shock and grief. Neither uniformly active nor passive, these shivers denote a mode of historical subjectivity that corresponds most closely to the middle voice, combining aspects of both agency and patiency (of acting and being acted upon), but being not reducible to either.[16]

Tryvoga, Enduring War

In the closing section, I want to bring into this discussion the affective modality of *tryvoga*, which seems to me as crucial to the sensorial, emotive, corporeal and 'nocturnal' moments of peoples' emergence in these war records. It is a recurring effect, through which the violence of war is registered by (and on) the body, and that comes close to 'dread' and 'horror', also carries other semantic connotations. The Slavic word *tryvoga* (Ukr. *тривога*) also invokes disquiet, trepidation, fear, anxiety, and a state of alertness and alarm.[17] Numerous diaries and dreams give accounts of affect or mood. *Tryvoga* is also the title of Eva Alvor's drawing (Image 3, p. 144). It depicts a naked and curled body of a man, grasping with both hands his head in what looks like an agonising gesture of unbearable pain, or perhaps in an attempt to silence overwhelming sounds or thoughts. The man is inscribed within a red figure that contrasts starkly with a protective (womb) structure: the shape has sharp, piercing edges and resembles a menacing bird of prey, a thorny bush, or a laceration caused by a tearing force. The background of the image is a nearly indecipherable handwriting, and the scribbles that invoke all-consuming, obsessive thoughts or tormenting words, and which the subject is unable to silence. What is striking about the image is that its 'containment logic' is reversed: the wound, rather than being depicted as a laceration *on* the skin, encloses the body; the scripted thoughts, rather than being presented as occurring *in* the mind, encompass the body and the wound. Through this reversed logic of containment, the image expresses the corporeal and psychic precarity of people in the face of violence. The affective intensity of dread and horror (*tryvoga*), so palpable in that image, signifies an experience that makes the protective structures (of a bomb shelter, but also those of the body) porous, injurable and destructible. The dynamism of Alvor's image makes the body gripped by *tryvoga* appear not as static (though neither is the figure moving), but, rather, as quivering and trembling.

The affective-corporeal modality of tremors or vibrations, which I have identified as a recurring motif in these narratives, is also present in the photographs, for example in the close-up of fingers and toes, and their embodied tension, in Anastasiia Markeliuk's images (Images 7.4, 7.5 and 7.6, pp. 177–179). There is a connection between bodily tremble or tremor and the effect of *tryvoga*. In contrast to the paralysed state of horror embodied as enforced stillness, 'stiffness' or 'petrification' (cf. Cavarero, 2009; Kordela, 2015), *tryvoga* manifests as a 'quasi-movement' of tremor or as *trepidation* (a useful term in this context in that it combines the condition of anxiety and dread with that of tremor or quiver).

Also, *tryvoga* has a temporal dimension, which is lost in the English translation as dread, disquiet, or alarm. It is that of an overpowering experience that is *extended in time*. Its symptomatic situation in the diaries, it seems to me, is that of a prolonged waiting in a bomb shelter, but there are also other moments of 'extended waiting' that the war enforces upon the people in the diaries—queuing for hours to a cash machine or a shop, waiting at a border, waiting in intensified traffic, etc. *Tryvoga* connotes that the dread, fear and alertness that register as bodily tremors are not a momentary occurrence, but a *lasting experience of pain*, which the subject comes to endure.

In concluding this chapter, I want to suggest that enduring or bearing the pain together, or rather *bearing each other in that lasting pain*, there emerges a situation of reciprocal holding (cf. Frosh, 2015). While the etymology of the word *tryvoga* is contested (see Nilsson, 1999), it has been suggested that it has a shared root with the verb 'to last', 'to stay put', 'to remain' (Ukr. *тривати*, Pl. *trwać*), and is related to the word 'tree' (PIE *deru-* meaning 'to be firm, solid and steadfast' (see 'Tree', n.d.)).[18] That quality endurance as *remaining in place*—as withstanding war—is a key characteristic of representing and imagining people in these archives. Stephen Frosh's theoretical account of endurance as relational ethics (2015) captures this connection between people and togetherness, or being-with and being-towards one another, as an unbearable, shattering experience that lies beyond the subject's control or initiation. Writing in a different context, but one that I think is applicable also here, Frosh suggests that the 'demand for endurance faces us with exposure to something that we cannot avoid; we just have to stay with it until it comes to an end' (2005, p. 171).

Finally, insofar as *tryvoga,* and shivering as its corporeal expressions, connote endurance of a long-lasting and painful experience, they also help understand better the role of the witness in these visual and narrative archives of war. Perhaps what they can help us understand better is the link between ethics and politics in witnessing more broadly. In continental philosophical scholarship on testimony (see Derrida, 2005; Felman & Laub, 1992; Oliver, 2001, 2015), testimonial ethics and politics are closely linked with the subject's (spatial-temporal) proximity to the traumatic event, and to the fact of their survival (even if they narrate is as a 'partial' or 'incomplete' survival, cf. Zolkos, 2010). Their survival subsequently forms a kind of ethical obligation (a call or 'appointment') to speak, listen and give testimony *in the place of* those who have not survived. Derrida (2005) thus argues that the testimonial speech act is a call to be believed that takes the spatial and temporal proximity to the catastrophic event as a condition of its possibility (every witness pleas, according to Derrida, 'believe me, I have been there, believe me, I have seen it'). The voices in the Ukrainian war diaries ask their listeners to critically reflect on how the relationality of endurance is understood in connection to the ethical and political demands of witnessing. 'Proximity' is not synonymous here with propinquitous location. Rather, it connotes the corporeal imprint (tremor, shiver) of intensive affects (*tryvoga*) in the emergence of political people, as both an affirmation of freedom and of relational ethics in the endurance of war.

Notes

1 I take the phrase 'open history' (to human bodies, effects and shivers) from Farge (2007).
2 I am indebted to Bohdan Shumylovych and Chari Larsson for their feedback on the earlier drafts of this chapter, and to Simone Drichel for conversations about ethics of endurance.

3 The phrase is used by Will Harris in Kaminsky, 2019.
4 That question recurs, partly, by way of resisting the denial of the independent existence of Ukrainian people in Russian war propaganda (e.g. Vladislav Surkov's claim that 'there is no such thing as Ukraine' (quoted in Düden, 2020)).
5 For a discussion of 'in spite of all' in Didi-Huberman's philosophy see Gustafsson, 2023.
6 This is not to idealise familial and other relations in the diaries. Friends, family, neighbours and strangers encountered in the shared spaces of the underground shelters are frequently depicted as sources of major frustration, resentment or anger (see e.g. Oksana V.'s diary, p. 85–86).
7 On 'waiting time' see Baraitser, 2017 and Salisbury and Baraitser, 2020, though the inertia of bodies in a bomb shelter is quite different from experiences of waiting in the mental health context.
8 The sound companion of the figure of underground shelter is the siren announcing an air alarm. It features as a strikingly ambiguous occurrence in the diaries; while for some it incites panic and anxiety (Daryna P., March 3, p. 245), a forceful awakening (Annamaria T., March 3, p. 244), and indexes an approaching threat (Anastasiia B., March 10, p. 199-200); it appeals to Mariana H.'s sister for whom it resembles 'the singing of whales, [their] way to confess love and establish mutual communication' (March 12, p. 209).
9 Mental and physical weariness are an important and recurring motif in many of the diaries as people report being tired of 'strong emotions' (Olha K., March 14, p. 46) and 'everyday overload' (Yelyzaveta B., April 7, p. 218), but often without any specific reason. Exhaustion can function as an all-pervasive state: 'I can't find the strength to work well, to read [and] study texts, or just fiction, to read anything that is not a news feed for the day. I have no power to respond to friends from abroad or elsewhere. I'm just really tired' (Olha K., March 27, p. 48). 'I'm so unnaturally tired – I am just a body', writes Stefaniia K. (April 5, p. 62). Fatigue signifies a profound systemic disorganisation of the self due to the stress and trauma of war (cf. Hunt, 2010, pp. 6–12).
10 An example of the 'fort-da' game in the diaries is found in Oksana D.'s excerpt (May 7, p. 96) where she identifies the switching on and off city lights (so as to obscure urban centres' location at night) with a 'fort-da' rhythm of 'now you see me, now you don't': 'Where is Ukraine?/*turns off the light*/There is no Ukraine/*turns on the lights*/Here is Ukraine!/*turns off the lights*/[...]'.
11 Arendt identifies kinship as the governing principle of a family, which she calls 'shelter and a mighty fortress in an inhospitable, alien world' (1993/2005, p. 94, modified); a depiction with which surely psychoanalysis and feminist criticism alike would have a quarrel with. The representations of family in *Diaries of War and Life* highlight the capacity of familial relations to be both a source of care and meaningful connections with others and to reverberate and amplify the violence of war (see e.g. Oksana V., March 20, 22 and 27, p. 86).
12 Emphasis in the original.
13 I thank Chari Larsson for this observation.
14 In personal communication, Bohdan Shumylovych has noted the future-oriented and anticipatory aspect of a shiver as a 'foreboding' or 'foreknowledge' of violence: 'the body [...] quivers in anticipation of violence, but once [the fighting] begins, the tremor subsides'.
15 Emphasis mine.
16 In *Margins of Philosophy* Derrida outlines the concept of *la différance* by invoking its comparison to the middle voice, of which he says that it is 'an operation that is not an operation'; the middle voice refers to what is unexplainable as either passion or agency, but, rather, a 'nontransivity' that

is repressed by the binary opposition of active and passive voice (1972/1982, pp. 9, 189).

17 In Oksana D.'s diary (p. 94), she calls her emergency bag, prepared for when she needs to evacuate to the bomb shelter, tryvozhna sumka, an 'alarm backpack' (also 'alarmed').

18 Quite a few drawings and dreams in *Diaries of War and Life* depict forests and trees, referencing (in my reading) questions of withstanding and enduring violence, as well as renewal and repair, and which cut across the arboreal and human register.

References

Arendt, H. (2005). Introduction into politics. In J. Kohn (Ed.), *The promise of politics* (pp. 93–200). Schocken Books. (Original work published in 1993)

Baraitser, L. (2017). *Enduring time*. Bloomsbury.

Bronfen, E. (2013). *Night passages: Philosophy, literature and film (E. Bronfen & D. Brenner, Trans.)*. Columbia University Press.

Cavarero, A. (2009). *Horrorism: Naming contemporary violence* (W. McCuaig, Trans.). Columbia University Press.

Derrida, J. (2005). Poetics and politics of witnessing (O. Pasanen, Trans.). In T. Dutoit & O. Pasanen (Eds.), *Sovereignties in question* (pp. 65–96). Fordham University Press.

Didi-Huberman, G. (2005). *Confronting images: Questioning the ends of a certain history of art* (J. Goodman, Trans.). The Pennsylvania State University Press. (Original work published 1990)

Didi-Huberman, G. (2016a). The render sensible (J. Gladding, Trans.). In A. Badiou, P. Bourdieu, J. Butler, G. Didi-Huberman, S. Khiari & J. Rancière (Eds.), *What is a people?* (pp. 65–86). Columbia University Press. (Original work published 2013)

Didi-Huberman, G. (2016b). *Uprisings*. Gallimard.

Didi-Huberman, G. (2018). *Survival of the fireflies* (L. S. Mitchell, Trans.). University of Minnesota Press. (Original work published 2008)

Didi-Huberman, G. (2019). Photo-papers (M. Wawrzyńczak, Trans.). In A. Duńczyk-Szulc (Ed.), *Dispersed contact. Photographers from the Ringelblum Archive: Reinterpreted* (pp. 8–41). Emanuel Ringelblum Historical Institute.

Farge, A. (2007). *Effusion et tourment, le récit des corps: Histoire du peuple au XVIIIe siècle*. Odile Jacob.

Felman, S. & Laub, D. (1992). *Testimony: Crises of witnessing in literature, psychoanalysis, and history*. Routledge.

Frosh, S. (2015). Endurance. *American Imago*, 72(2), 157–175.

Gustafsson, H. (2023). In spite of all (malgré tout). In M. Zolkos (Ed.), *The Didi-Huberman dictionary* (pp. 122–125). Edinburgh University Press.

Hunt, N. C. (2010). *Memory, war and trauma*. Cambridge University Press.

Kaminsky, I. (2019). *Deaf republic*. Faber & Faber.

Klein, I. (Host). (2022, March 15). Ezra Klein interviews Timothy Snyder [Audio podcast transcript]. In *The Ezra Klein Show*. https://www.nytimes.com/2022/03/15/podcasts/transcript-ezra-klein-interviews-timothy-snyder.html

Kordela, A. K. (2015, October 3). Horror. In *Political concepts: A lexicon*. https://www.politicalconcepts.org/horror-kiarina-kordela/

Oliver, K. (2001). *Witnessing: Beyond recognition*. University of Minnesota Press.

Oliver, K. (2015). Witnessing, recognition, and response ethics. *Philosophy & Rhetoric*, *48*(4), 473–493.

Nilsson, T. K. (1999). An old Polish sound law and the etymology of Polish trwoga and trwać and Russian trevóga. *Historische Sprachforschung/Historical Linguistics*, *112*, 143–159.

Renan, E. (2018). What is a nation? (M. F. N. Giglioli, Trans.) In M. F. N. Giglioli (Ed.), *What is a nation? and other political writings* (pp. 247–263). Columbia University Press. (Original work published 1882)

Rosanvallon, P. (1998). *Le Peuple introuvable: Histoire de la représentation démocratique en France*. Folio Histoire.

Salisbury, L. & L. Baraitser. (2020). Depressing time: Waiting, melancholia, and the psychoanalytic practice of care. In E. Kirtsoglou & B. Simpson (Eds.), *The time of anthropology: Studies of contemporary chronopolitics* (pp. 103–121). Routledge.

Snyder, T. (2022, September 6). Ukraine holds the future: The war between democracy and nihilism. *Foreign Affairs*. https://www.foreignaffairs.com/ukraine/ukraine-war-democracy-nihilism-timothy-snyder?check_logged_in=1&utm_medium=promo_email&utm_source=lo_flows&utm_campaign=registered_user_welcome&utm_term=email_1&utm_content=20230824

'Tree'. (n.d.). *Online etymology dictionary [website]*. https://www.etymonline.com/search?q=tree

Winnicott, D. (1953). Transitional objects and transitional phenomena: A study of the first Not-Me possession. *The International Journal of Psychoanalysis, 1953, 34*, 89–97.

Zolkos, M. (2010). *Reconciling community and subjective life: Trauma testimony as political theorising in the work of Jean Améry and Imre Kertész*. Bloomsbury.

INDEX

Affect 1, 2, 4, 5, 121, 171, 276, 277, 282, 283; *see also* emotions
Anger 3, 5, 38, 40, 41, 104, 105, 106, 109, 115, 251, 253, 254, 255, 256, 257, 259, 260n2, 270, 284n6
Anxiety 3, 4, 6, 11, 14, 16, 19, 23, 37, 38, 39, 104, 106, 108, 109, 134, 137, 138, 253, 254, 258, 259, 279, 281, 282, 284n8; *see also* tryvoga
Aristotle 252

Benjamin, Jessica 108
Benveniste, Émile 163, 171
Beradt, Charlotte 269, 270
Bion, Wilfred 111
Body 3, 5, 6, 11, 12, 13, 14, 15, 16, 17, 18, 19, 26, 39, 42, 104, 118, 124, 125, 126, 135, 256, 266, 267, 268, 269, 270, 277, 280, 281, 282, 284n9, 284n14; shivering 6, 274, 280, 281, 283
Breath 15, 42, 103; and breathlessness 102, 103
Butler, Judith 108, 110, 118

Care 5, 15, 36, 38, 102, 104, 169, 172, 251, 275, 276, 284n11
Cognition 12, 13
Community 7, 24, 32, 127, 128, 165, 172, 251, 253, 277, 279; national 24
Consciousness 2, 11, 12, 15, 31, 33, 110, 113, 121, 164; phenomenology of 2, 11

Contemplation 14
Contemplative studies 2, 14, 15, 16
Courage 5, 19, 33, 34, 40, 113, 251, 252, 253, 254, 259, 260,265, 278
Crépon, Marc 5, 251, 256

Death drive 4, 111, 112
Depressive anxiety 4
Depressive position 108, 114; *see also* Klein, Melanie
Derrida, Jacques 1, 4, 131, 132, 133, 134, 135, 139, 140n2, 141n10, 283, 284n16; and image philosophy 4, 131, 132, 133, 134, 135; *see also* ruins
Diaries of War and Life (project) 3, 5, 26, 117, 119, 126, 128, 162, 163, 164, 165, 166, 169, 171, 172, 261, 263, 274, 275, 276, 277, 278, 279, 280, 284n11, 285n18
Diary-writing 1–2, 11–21, 22–24, 26–28, 31–34, 39–40, 41–42, 126–129, 251–252, 261–272; and hope 19, 34; as a space of safety 19; and war 11, 19, 25–26, 29, 39–40, 121–122, 128–129
Didi-Huberman, Georges 3, 6, 7, 27, 275, 276, 277, 279, 280, 284n5
Drawings 2, 4, 12, 19, 26, 27, 37, 131, 132, 133, 135, 137,139, 140, 285n18
Dread; *see tryvoga*

Dreams 3, 5, 6, 17, 18, 19, 26, 27, 28, 31, 32, 34, 101, 103, 104, 106, 109, 110, 111, 112, 113, 114, 138, 251, 261, 266, 267, 268, 269, 270, 271, 275, 276, 278, 281, 285n18; proleptic 31
Dreamscape 3, 101, 113, 114
Dumka 5, 261, 272

Ego-documentation 1, 2; *see also* Presser, Jacques
Ego-narration; *see* Ego-documentation
Embodiment 5, 13, 17, 26
Emotions 3, 5, 12, 15, 17, 18, 23, 33, 37, 38, 39, 40, 41, 135, 137, 138, 251, 252, 253, 254, 255, 257, 258, 259, 278, 279, 280, 284n9; hiding and control of 258; and resistance 5, 251, 252, 253, 255, 256, 259, 260; undermining 255
Endurance 2, 5, 6, 7, 26, 251, 274, 279, 283, 283n2
Evil 135, 136, 137, 141n6, 141n7, 260n2
Exhaustion 41, 42, 102, 106, 256, 277, 284n9; *see also* fatigue
Experience 1, 2, 3, 5, 6, 11, 12, 13, 14, 15, 16, 17, 18, 19, 24, 25, 26, 27, 28, 29, 30, 31, 33, 37, 38, 39, 40, 102, 103, 107, 108, 109, 110, 112, 117, 118, 119, 120, 121, 122, 123, 124, 125, 126, 128, 132, 138, 139, 140, 163, 164, 165, 167, 168, 170, 254, 257, 258, 259, 264, 266, 269, 277, 278, 279, 280, 281, 282, 283, 284n7; embodied 13, 16, 19, 26, 29, 120; lived 1, 2, 3, 28, 140, 164; singular 24, 139; subjective 2, 13, 14, 24, 102

Fatigue 41, 169, 277, 284n9; *see also* exhaustion
Fear 3, 16, 25, 31, 38, 40, 104, 105, 106, 108, 109, 110, 113, 125, 128, 135, 252, 253, 254, 255, 257, 258, 259, 270, 274, 276, 278, 279, 280, 281, 282
Fireflies 3, 32
Flowers 131, 132
Freedom 6, 7, 33, 253, 274, 275, 276, 283
Freud, Sigmund 107, 108, 109, 110, 111, 112, 113, 275, 277; *see also* psychoanalysis
Friendship 5, 171, 251

Fright 108, 109, 118; *see also tryvoga*

Gratitude 5, 42, 251, 255, 278
Guilt 3, 38, 41, 114, 115, 258

Honesty 39, 279
Hope 5, 6, 19, 32, 34, 103, 107, 110, 111, 114, 122, 251, 252, 254, 257, 258, 260n4, 267, 268; loss of 111, 260n4

Images; *see* drawings; photography; war photography; war paintings
Imagination 1, 17, 18, 27, 121, 129
Imperialism 30
Irony 4

Joy 5, 24, 34, 38, 118, 251, 253, 254, 259, 266, 279

Kant, Immanuel 28, 136, 141n7
Klein, Melanie 108, 112, 114
Koselleck, Reinhard 28

Language 13, 14, 16, 19, 23, 24, 29, 30, 111, 121, 127, 128, 135, 139, 171, 253, 265, 266; remaining 125, 279, 283
Loss 2, 4, 41, 105, 107, 108, 109, 110, 111, 113, 118, 120, 123, 124, 132, 135, 140, 251, 254, 255, 260n4, 274; of identity 124
Love 5, 110, 118, 126, 141n9, 251, 253, 254, 259, 275, 284n8

Meditation 2, 11, 14, 15, 16, 17, 18, 19, 24, 257
Melancholia 4, 107, 108, 110, 111, 115
Memory 1, 3, 4, 5, 12, 17, 19, 24, 27, 28, 29, 107, 110, 119, 132, 134, 261, 263, 266, 267, 269; collective 3, 24, 28, 29, 263
Mourning 4, 24, 107, 108, 110, 111, 113, 120, 165, 169, 255, 264
Mutism 3, 23, 37

Paintings 4, 19, 27, 140n6, 141n6
Paranoid-schizoid position 114; *see also* Klein, Melanie
Pasolini, Pier Paolo 3, 32
People 1, 3, 4, 6, 7, 11, 12, 13, 16, 19, 22, 23, 24, 25, 27, 28, 30, 31, 32, 34, 37, 38, 39, 40, 41, 105, 106, 109, 113, 114, 117, 120, 122, 131, 132,

134, 137, 138, 163, 166, 168, 169, 172, 251, 253, 254, 255, 256, 259, 262, 263, 264, 265, 266, 269, 270, 271, 272, 274, 275, 276, 277, 278, 279, 280, 282, 283, 284n4, 284n9; nocturnal 6, 276, 279; political 6, 274, 275, 276, 277, 279, 280, 283
Photography 4, 5, 162, 163, 164, 165, 166, 168, 169, 170, 171, 172; vernacular 4, 163, 166, 170, 171, 172; and war 5, 163, 164, 165, 172; see also photojournalism
Photojournalism 5, 165, 169, 170; see also photography
Precarious 127
Presser, Jacques 27; see also ego-documentation
Psychoanalysis 107, 108, 109, 114, 115, 164, 284n11; and war 107; see also Freud, Sigmund

Quiet trauma 3, 4, 5, 162, 165, 169, 172

Renan, Ernest 24, 274
Reparation 4, 114, 115
Resistance 2, 3, 5, 7, 29, 33, 34, 110, 126, 129, 167, 251, 252, 253, 255, 256, 259, 260, 261, 262, 263, 264, 265, 267, 268, 269, 271, 272n4, 274, 275, 276, 279
Responsibility 3, 5, 34, 114, 164, 172, 261
Roth, Harold 2, 14, 15
Ruins 3, 4, 110, 118, 131, 132, 133, 134, 135, 137, 138, 139, 140, 276; as psychic devastation 4; see also Derrida, Jacques
Rupture 1, 3, 4, 117, 118, 120, 121, 122, 123, 125, 126, 127, 129

Sartre, Jean-Paul 33, 269
Shame 3, 38, 40, 41, 258
Shelter 2, 6, 12, 17, 22, 25, 104, 113, 125, 134, 137, 141n9, 168, 269, 276, 277, 281, 282, 284n6, 284n7, 284n8, 284n11, 285n17
Shiver; see body shivering
Shock 22, 23, 38, 109, 118, 164, 259, 281
Silence 3, 37, 39, 102, 111, 262, 282; internal 3; see also mutism
Sirens 101, 102, 103, 104, 109, 111, 112, 115, 125

Snyder, Timothy 253, 274, 275, 276
Solidarity 2, 5, 6, 7, 34, 105, 132, 251, 253, 255, 269, 271, 274, 275, 278
Spectator 134, 137, 139, 162, 163, 166, 167, 168, 169, 171
Spectatorship 163, 169, 171, 172; as friendship 163; see also testimony; witnessing
Subjective experience; see lived experience
Survival 7, 26, 119,122, 126, 137, 283

Testimony 5, 6, 164, 274, 283; see also witnessing
Time 3, 4, 6, 12, 16, 17, 19, 23, 24, 25, 26, 27, 28, 30, 31, 32, 33, 34, 36, 37, 39, 41, 42, 103, 104, 106, 107, 110, 111, 113, 115, 117, 118, 119, 119, 120, 121, 123, 124, 125, 126, 127, 129, 131, 133, 136, 138, 139, 140, 141n10, 162, 164, 167, 169, 252, 253, 254, 255, 256, 259, 261, 262, 263, 265, 266, 268, 269, 270, 272, 276, 277, 280, 281, 282, 284n7
Trauma 3, 4, 5, 12, 15, 18, 33, 38, 104, 109, 110, 111, 112, 113, 115, 125, 127, 137, 138, 139, 141n10, 162, 163, 164, 165, 169, 170, 172, 276, 284n9; theory of 164; unassimilable 164; see also quiet trauma
Truth 22, 27, 104, 111, 114, 129, 133, 140, 166, 171
Truthfulness 22, 27, 31
Tryvoga 6, 144, 274, 281, 282, 283; see also fright
Two Months of War (project); see Diaries of War and Life (project)

Ukraine 1–2, 22–23, 24, 131–132, 167–168, 271–272, 274–276; the full-scale invasion of 1–2, 11, 22–23, 107, 117–118, 119, 131–132, 137–138, 140, 163–164, 165, 274–276; post-colonial theory and 30
Unconscious 1, 28, 31, 112, 118, 121, 123, 124, 126, 127, 129, 138, 277

Violence 1, 2, 3, 5, 6, 7, 32, 33, 34, 105, 108, 110, 111, 114, 115, 121, 123, 128, 131, 138, 166, 168, 251, 256, 274, 280, 281, 282, 284n11, 284n14, 285n18; see also war

War 1–2, 11, 25–26, 31, 32–33, 101–102, 107–108, 117–129, 131, 137–138, 163–168, 262–263, 271–272, 279–283; collective memory and 28–29, 140; diary-writing inresponse to 11, 19, 25–26, 29, 39–40, 121–122, 128–129; enduring 25–26, 281–283; lived experience of 1, 2, 3, 28, 140, 164; psycho-social perspectives on 1–2, 11, 15–18, 31, 32–34, 37–42, 101–114, 117–129, 279–283; sounds of 101, 111, 112, 115, 117–118, 125; subjective experience of 2, 13, 14, 24, 102

War Diaries (project); *see Diaries of War and Life* (project)

Witnessing 1, 6, 131, 138, 139, 164, 169, 172, 283; *see also* testimony

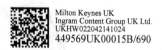
Milton Keynes UK
Ingram Content Group UK Ltd.
UKHW022042141024
449569UK00015B/690